INTUITIVE EATING

12 Principles for Healthy Mindful Eating Habits: A Revolutionary Non-Diet Workbook Program To Unlock Your Mind And Stop Emotional and Binge Eating

Ashley Brain

Table of Contents

Introduction

Modern standards of beauty are ruthless: "beautiful" means "thin." Trying to meet these standards, millions of men and women are chronically plagued by diets and torn in gyms. This method of losing weight has a beginning, but no end: in order to keep fit, you need to limit yourself more in food and increase physical activity. You can't stop - you will gain weight. The price of such a lifestyle is food "breakdowns" when a huge amount of "forbidden" foods are eaten overnight and the "yo-yo effect" when weight is either gained or lost. The "escort group" is unstable self-esteem, especially bodily, depression, anxiety disorders. Food, instead of one of the pleasures of life, becomes a source of constant and tremendous tension.

However, food is the very first metaphor of love, the very first relationship that a born person builds. When a child falls, he immediately receives food, warmth, protection, and love. That is why violations of relations with food always force one to look at other relations in a person's life - with a partner, friends, children, parents, but most importantly - at relations with oneself. Strongly coarsening, we can say that the root of eating disorders is the violation of relations with oneself, in the inability to love and accept oneself.

There is no need for violence and eternal control over yourself in order to overcome this problem: you just need to learn to trust yourself.

The question that always arises in many people: can I lose weight by giving up diets and switching to intuitive nutrition? To predict how events will develop for you personally,

Try to answer the following questions:
1. How often do you continue to eat after the feeling of comfortable satiation has already come?
2. Do you often overeat before you go on a new diet (realizing that you can't afford to eat all this for a long time on a diet)?
3. Do you have time to cope with emotions or overcome boredom?
4. Do you relate to those who steadily dislike physical activity?
5. Do you exercise only when you are on a diet?
6. Do you often happen to skip a meal or eat only when you literally fall from hunger, and as a result, you overeat?
7. Do you feel guilty if you overeat or eat "unhealthy food," which ultimately leads to even more overeating (all the same, everything has already disappeared)?

If you answered "yes" to all or some of these questions, your current weight might be higher than your physiological weight, which your body has programmed to maintain on its own from birth, without any additional effort on your part. It is very likely that you are able to return to this weight as a result of the transition to intuitive nutrition. The most important thing to remember: weight loss should not be an end in itself, because switching to an intuitive diet for weight loss will greatly interfere with the development of your ability to listen to the body's internal signals.

Chapter 1: The First Principle - Unlearning the Dieting Mindset

In the ranks of those who are losing weight, the legend is widespread that there is one single, treasured, almost especially designed-for-you diet. If you find it, then the problem of losing weight is solved forever. This sacred diet is easy to follow - it is perceived as comfortable, and you simply don't notice any prohibitions. You lose weight on it remarkably quickly and feel great. You can stick to it all your life. It's just as difficult to find it as the Holy Grail - in search; you will have to try on yourself all the achievements of dietary thought...

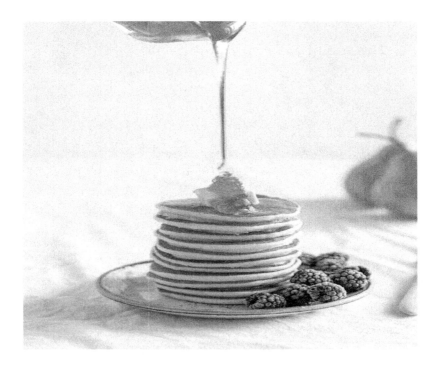

This myth is based on a simple medical fact: about 5-10% of people in a population are able to withstand significant restrictions on the variety and calorie intake of food for a long time, and therefore, keep weight loss as a result of dietary behavior for a long time. These 5–10% primarily include people with a healthy, undisturbed type of food, genetically prone to maintaining low body weight effortlessly.

A healthy type of food we call the ability to listen to the internal signals of hunger and satiety and choose food according to internal needs, and not considerations of calorie content, "benefit" / "harm," belonging to a group of proteins or carbohydrates.

When you begin to talk about intuitive nutrition in a lecture, exclamations are surely heard: "My husband eats exactly that!" "My aunt always ate like that," "I didn't know that I was an intuitive eater." After asking in more detail, you find that the aforementioned husband and aunt had no problems with either self-esteem or weight - they were not necessarily thin at all and did not cause discomfort, and they always ate exactly as much as they wanted, - no more and no less. These are natural, natural, intuitive eaters, people whose eating behavior could not be spoiled by parents, mass media, and general dietary madness. If such people are "transplanted" to food with certain restrictions, they will calmly, with significant suffering, endure this period, and then they will be able to maintain their reduced weight for a short time. Usually, the situation unfolds in a completely different way: sooner or later, the diet is followed by a "breakdown," after which the motivation to continue following it is greatly reduced. "This one doesn't seem to help," we think, "it's probably not for me, I'll look for something else." The new diet system causes a surge of motivation, hope, and desire, this time guaranteed to succeed. It lasts for a while, then the cycle repeats...

Seeking to lose weight, as if enchanted, he is looking for "his own diet," over and over again trying new ones - those that are now in fashion, or those that have succeeded in succeeding for someone else. However, the truth is that "working" for you personally - any diet. Yes, you heard right, and there is no typo here. Absolutely any of the existing nutrition systems focused on weight loss, sooner or later lead to a result. The differences are minimal. Why? Because the goal of any diet is to change your current nutrition system and make the body get rid of a certain amount of kilograms. Any restriction of fats and simple carbohydrates (namely, almost any existing diet is built on this) achieves this goal. It's important not to forget that...

... In fact. Any diet works. Temporarily

You choose a diet that promises rapid weight loss in a short time. We call fast weight loss of more than 1-1.5 kg per week. You gain courage, tragically bite your 4 crackers with a glass of yogurt a day, and at night you have dreams about chocolate muffins. You are constantly tormented by hunger, your body catastrophically lacks vitamins and minerals (vitamins in the pharmacy that is vitamin complexes are not only very little absorbed but can be toxic), in addition, you are dehydrated, because fast diets often include a component of active excretion of fluid from the body, and drink the prescribed liter of water per day. But, most importantly, the brain receives a distinct signal from the digestive system: "Attention! Turn on the hungry regime!" The human brain is little familiar with the modern cult of excessive thinness and still thinks caveman.

In addition to the symptoms of lethargy, drowsiness, unwillingness to start any action, especially implying physical activity known to everyone who has ever been on a strict diet (another minus is that it simply does not work to make regular motor activity an inseparable part of his life). It also includes the symptom of "holding" any calories that accidentally wandered into the body. In other words, everything that can be converted to fat is converted to fat. In the "hungry mode," other important changes occur with the body - for example, the number of enzymes producing fat cells doubles.

Our body perceives hunger as a serious threat and prepares "heavy artillery" in order to reliably survive the next hunger period.

Therefore, sitting on a diet, you decide not to lose weight, but to gain weight, simply after a brief period of a more "harmonious" life.

But what about that 5-10 %, you ask? Why aren't they getting better? Do their physiological mechanisms regulate their body? Of course not. What is the difference then? The difference is that these people hear the internal signals of the body, telling them when and how they need to eat, and at the same time, they are genetically not inclined to fullness.

Any restriction in food gives us a completely natural resistance, both physiological - the body strives to suck in any available calories and put them in reserve for a rainy day - and psychological. A person on a diet is irritable, sad, and unhappy. He fights all the time with temptations, and he always confronts the devilish voices that ask for "well, that cookie."

It is human nature to have an extremely negative attitude to any restrictions - this is one of the basic properties of the human psyche. That is why, as a punishment for the violation of freedom, mankind came up with a conclusion - restriction of freedom.

Before I began to study nutritional dependencies, I devoted many years to working with chemical addictions, mainly drug addiction. When I worked in a men's prison and wrote my notes about the life of male prisoners who use drugs, I often came across an indignant reaction: "In such good conditions, a prison is not a punishment!" Under good conditions, it was meant respectful human attitude on the part of the staff, access to medical help and education, decent conditions (a small cell-room for one person with a bathroom), and hot food. My interlocutors did not have experience of imprisonment, and it was rather difficult for me to explain that all these buns are not worth the simple fact that the territory is surrounded by gates, beyond which it will be impossible for several more years. And that people in such conditions should feel bad, very bad.

Do you know what the prisoner's favorite TV show is? The series "Prison Break."

Diet is your personal prison, and you will definitely want to break out of it by all means. The "prisoner" will be torn to "freedom," to treasured carbohydrates and fats, to overeat them, because this is the "last time," and then again locked up. And so - an infinite number of cycles. The emergence of a new diet renews a fairly dull motivation and adds faith in one's own strength - the effect of novelty is triggered. (The most "faithful" guardians of the program in the obesity treatment clinic are the patients of the first three months. They have the most intense dynamics of weight loss. After three months, novelty and pride in the taken step fade, maintaining motivation becomes more difficult after 6 months, and the novelty disappears altogether, there is a crisis of motivation).

It's not without reason that the clinic in which I started working with overeating therapy, where the average BMI is 42 (this means very large excess weight, people with such a BMI weigh 110–120 kg or more, depending on height), is full of people who know much more than me about all existing diets - they tried them all. There is a special term in dietetics - "yo-yo effect." Yo-yo is a Japanese children's toy, a wheel rising and falling along a rope. As a figure on the scales of endless diet victims.

Myth - Nutrition Must Be Monitored, Otherwise You Will Immediately Get Fat

When I talk about the intuitive nutrition approach and mention that it implies a complete rejection of any restrictions, there is always a person who asks: "Without diets? But how then do you watch your diet? "And I will answer that I do not follow my diet because I do not suspect him of anything.

In every joke, as you know, there is a fraction of a joke. The word "follow" reflects the activity of the paranoid part of the personality - the one that feels suspicious and distrust, the one that absolutely does not believe that the one who needs to be "watched" is capable of something good on its own and correct. Each of us has a paranoid part of our personality; healthy distrust does not allow us to let young children go alone in an unfamiliar place and leave the door to the house wide open in our absence. However, with regard to food, paranoia has long since become widespread and has crossed the boundaries of a healthy reaction.

The diet industry has succeeded - the idea of the need for nutrition control has become widespread. The vast majority of people are convinced that if they do not count calories, items, choose low-fat products in the store, and they will immediately turn into a swollen, thickened, ugly semblance of themselves. So, in Miyazaki's famous animated film "Spirited Away," the Chihiro girls, found themselves in an enchanted amusement park inhabited by ghosts and unable to deny themselves delicious food laid out in a street cafe, suddenly turn into fat, continuously chewing pigs.

As a result, most people are in a situation of constant restrictions, more severe when they are "on a diet," and less severe in a non-dietary period.

A catastrophic distrust of one's own body and its capabilities is formed to make an adequate choice of the right food at any given moment. The phrases "I'm hungry," "I would like to eat this ...," "I am very hungry," "not very hungry" are gradually disappearing from our speech, but we very often say "I need to eat," "I should not eat this cake" and even "I absolutely cannot eat sweets." The phrase "good appetite" sounds like a curse, although a few decades ago, it was a characteristic of a healthy, full of human strength.

In fact, our body is capable of doing this work without our participation.

The body has the original wisdom, allowing it to select what you need to eat now and to know how much it needs to be eaten. The trouble is that we are accustomed to invade these natural settings from birth, feeding children not according to their needs, but in accordance with the current position of pediatricians and children's nutritionists on this issue.

If you return to the body the opportunity to choose, hear the voice of your own needs, stop when satiety is reached, then the need to monitor nutrition will disappear by itself. The body will do this work for you, and will do it much more efficiently than you.

Chapter 2: The Second Principle – Make Peace with Food for Good

The beginning of a new diet very often means an attempt (most often not the first and not the only one) to start a new life, that is, to change the existing course of things for the better. Most often, these attempts end in complete failure. Why is this happening? Why can't we solve our own problems with diet? And here is why...

When you go on a diet, you are not setting the goal that can be achieved with it. Your goal is to change your life, and for this, you need to lose weight permanently. Forever become minus five, ten, twenty-eight - underline the necessary - kilograms, and - find a new job, meet your love, decide to have a baby, change relationships with parents - underline the necessary. No diet can achieve this goal.

Losing weight on purpose is not necessary at all. It is enough to change your own eating behavior, and the weight normalizes by itself.

But why do you need this? Really, what an idiotic question. To look good. I'll look good - I'll be glad when I see myself in the mirror, I will become more confident, I'm proud of my walk, I'm in a good mood right now, I will want new dresses, men will be crazy for me ... and then my problems with love, work and relationships will be finally solved!

This is a monstrously pathological installation, although it is usually used. Why is she wrong? Because of the fragile foundation of your own appearance (more precisely, your own assessment of it), you are building a building of your whole life. At the very first serious failure in life - dismissal, disagreement with a partner - you do not need to take care of the fragile crystal of your beauty more - anyway, "chef, everything is gone, gone!". What are you doing? Right, enter into an unnatural relationship with a busy group of cakes. And more than once. Or, say, with a five-story cake. The motivation to reduce and stabilize your weight can only be internal: I want this, I need it. Inner and no more.

In fact. Clearly articulate goals. Separate life change from food change.

... I am losing weight because it is important for me to be healthy. Why should I be healthy? To live longer, have time to do more, have time to meet your love or enjoy the existing, see, and educate grandchildren.

... I want to be active. I want to fly to Australia or go to the Carpathians. I want to climb the Eiffel Tower or Mount Sokol in the Crimea. I want to teach my daughter to jump rope. By the way, I want to give birth to this very daughter.

... I want to feel good. Easy and free. Move smoothly and feminine.

These are examples of internal, true motivation for losing weight. What you can "buy" for your new body - the attention of representatives of the opposite sex, additional self-confidence - can be a pleasant bonus, but it cannot be the ultimate goal. The personal changes that you hope to achieve with the new body must be achieved before or during the process of losing weight. And then you will not need to lose weight at all - you simply will not notice the process of changes, they will occur naturally.

This requires an understanding of what really needs to change in your life. The relationship with food and the psychological role that food plays in your life. Separation of weight loss as a change in weight and body size from solving problems of professional unfulfillment, loneliness, fear of becoming a parent, or broken relationships with one's loved ones. This can be achieved not through diet, but by working on changing the image of the body and sustainable patterns of behavior, including food. For this, this book was written. Do you need a diet in this case? No, the diet actively interferes with this process, replacing the work of rebuilding life with the activity of replacing some foods in your diet with others. The real problems are the whole time it takes you to count calories.

Diet and Weight Loss Will Make Me Healthier

One of the most persistent and destructive misconceptions: a diet is necessary for healing the body! I'll be so healthy! People are stubbornly convinced that complete weights mean sick, and literally refuse to believe their eyes, if medical statistics are shown to the contrary.

The demonization of completeness as a symbol of literally all serious illnesses in the world had clear economic reasons: insurance companies needed a clear criterion by which it was possible to increase insurance premiums or refuse health insurance. Inevitably and symmetrically, thinness, for centuries symbolizing poverty, poor health, and ill-temper, suddenly became a sign of total health and economic viability.

In fact, as mentioned above, dietary experience forces the body to go into intensive production and storage of fat as soon as the period of dietary restrictions ends. Low-calorie diets double the amount of enzymes that produce and store fat. But this is far from the only change.

Evelyn Tribble, in the book Intuitive Nutrition, lists many of the negative health effects of a diet. In studies conducted both in rats and in humans, it was shown that dietary experience consistently reduces the intensity of losing weight with each new dietary attempt. This is well known to all experienced "thinners": the first dietary attempt is usually tolerated relatively easily and leads to a brilliant result - the loss of 8-10 kilograms is not uncommon. You rejoice and believe that you managed to avoid the fate of those who unsuccessfully go on diets and are not able to not only reduce but even maintain their existing weight. After a while, when the nasty excess weight is gaining again, it upsets you, but does not scare you - you know what to do. You go to the store for a special set of products and join the battle from Monday. This time, the results will probably be a little worse, and transferring the diet will be somewhat more difficult, but by the end of the prescribed minimum period, you can still easily change the size of your clothes to a smaller one. This may continue for several cycles until, finally, one day, you will find that the usual tool no longer works. You regularly live half-starving, earnestly complying with everything prescribed, but the weight does not move. You fall into despair, start looking for new methods, but other diets do not work either. In complete frustration, you begin to think about slimming teas, laxative pills, and ... find yourself in one step from the development of eating disorders, which will be discussed later.

In other words, the more active your dietary attempts are, the more often you will find yourself in a situation where you "cannot resist" so as not to eat something, and are not able to stop when you start eating. Diet really changes your eating behavior, only it changes it - for the worse, in the direction of disrupting a healthy type of diet.

The chronic experience of diets changes the shape of the body. And again, not in the direction we would like to! Those who constantly lose and gain weight, even in small volumes, tend to put off fat in the abdominal region - around the waist. This type of obesity is statistically associated with a risk of cardiovascular disease. Not surprisingly, a study of more than 3 thousand men and women, known as the Framingham Heart Pathology Study, which lasted 32 years, showed that, regardless of the initial weight, whether the subjects were thin or obese, regardless other cardiovascular risk factors (smoking, physical inactivity), those whose weight is constantly changing (yo-yo effect), are twice as likely to die from cardiovascular diseases, their mortality rate is much higher.

A study of the health of Harvard graduates showed that those who lose and again gain at least 5 kilograms over 10 years live less than those who maintain a stable weight. Psychological studies of the consequences of the dietary experience have shown that those who, in their teens, use the diet to regulate weight, are subsequently 8 times more likely to suffer from eating disorders. Diets significantly reduce self-confidence and self-esteem and forever associate your nutritional experience, not with the pleasure of satiety and the enjoyment of different tastes, but with a feeling of guilt for what you eat. Diets weaken, rather than reinforce, a sense of control over one's own eating behavior - even the illusory experience of eating forbidden foods (for example, if in an experiment the subject was offered food or a drink described as high-calorie, although in fact its calorie content was small) significantly increases the risk of food failure.

But that is not all. Most diets are based on a strong restriction of the products of one group - carbohydrates, fats, or both, in favor of products of another group, most often proteins. Both the Atkins diet, and the Dukan Diet, and the nutrition used by people who are actively "building" the body in the gym are based on high protein content. Weight loss on such a diet is really happening rapidly. But this is not the only change that needs to happen to your body. Excess protein causes increased growth and, as a result, increased aging. Protein molecules tend to "stick together" in red blood cells, reducing vascular patency, which causes an increased risk of:

- Alzheimer's disease;
- Parkinson's disease;
- amyloidosis;
- The general aging of internal organs.

Increased meat consumption leads to

- increased chance of osteoporosis;
- increased load on the liver and kidneys;
- increased risk of cancer;

- impaired digestion in the intestines;
- Undigested proteins activate the immune system, leading to autoimmune diseases.

Diets are a commercial product with very well done marketing. They sell hope for a better life, and in case of failure, they "switch arrows" to the buyer.

Nothing more successful in the commercial industry has been invented to this day. You can imagine that the support service of a software development company, where you contacted about the fact that the program you purchased is working with errors, tells you: you were not able to use it correctly, that's why the program is "buggy"! It is unlikely that such a company would have existed in the market for a long time. If you buy a new car and the air conditioner fails in it, or the headlight does not work, - well, it's your own fault, why did you breathe so much, why did you go in the heat? It is unlikely that any of us would think of saying in these cases - well, it's my fault, I haven't shown enough patience, I haven't learned to put up with mistakes. Why are we less careful with our bodies and, more importantly, with our own self-esteem than with our computer or machine?

The only case when the use of a diet is necessary and improves the quality of life is if the doctors find you have a medical condition in which some products cause you real physical damage. Allergies, celiac disease, autism - there are not so many such diseases. In all other cases, the only healthy way to establish a relationship with food and to avoid overeating is to give up all diets permanently.

I know that it sounds scary to you; it seems like a path to chaos and perpetual obesity. However, switching to an intuitive diet and living for some time in the body of an intuitive eater, you will find that unconsciously, without making any effort, you often choose to eat as prescribed by the best nutritionists. You will often want carbohydrates in the morning, because you don't like the heaviness in the stomach that appears from them in the evening, many store sweets will seem cloying, although you have not limited yourself to sweets for a day, many of you will feel the need to refuse meat - it just starts to seem tasteless. You will start to eat up much less food.

What is the problem then, you say, if dietary rules are not so bad, then why should they be discarded? Because any violent introduction of good and beneficial causes a human being to resist and attack naturally. Remember that it is enough for someone from your closest good intentions to tell you: "You should not eat this cake ...." like you, in the darkest mood, eat up the third piece. As part of an intuitive diet, there are no initial rules - you set the rules yourself, choosing only those that really work to improve your well-being. What we see as free choice does not cause resistance; we don't even notice that we are "observing" something.

At the same time, there may be no external differences between an intuitive eater and a professional fighter on the diet front - each of them can eat those products that we automatically consider "healthy and healthy," and what we consider "tasty, but harmful." The difference in approach, in the sensations from this food, in thoughts about it.

Intuitive Eater

Oh, I'm hungry! What do I want now? It's so hot. I want a cool, fresh ... probably sour or brackish... (looks in the refrigerator). Cottage cheese! Chopped Parsley! Exactly what is needed! (Imagines how he will feel when he eats.) It seems that this is not enough. I want to add something ... Warm, crispy ... Toast! (He makes a toast, spreads cottage cheese on it and eats it with appetite.) Mmm, how delicious! Got enough? It seems like something else ... Now sweet. Biscuits! (He eats cookies, drinks tea, thinking and listening to himself, eats another and gets up from the table contented and calm.)

Someone on a Diet

Two in the afternoon, I have to eat. What can I do now? (It is checked with a list or diagram.) You can curd with greens and a slice of bread. On the table is a cookie. Tasty, I guess. I want some cookies. You can't bear it. Otherwise, your ass will never fit into jeans. Cottage cheese is sick. I want sweets. Okay, there's nothing to do. (With a sigh, he makes cottage cheese with greens, adds a piece of bread, and chews sluggishly and without enthusiasm.) Come on! Cheer up! Look, what a fellow you are - didn't break anything! Clever and future slender beauty! As soon as you lose weight, let's go with you to the store and buy a dress. No, two dresses. Or three. I want some cookies. Why the hell should I limit myself when a huge number of people eat everything they want, and nothing happens for them?! Why?! Lord, for what?! By the way, since I was so smart today, can I afford one cookie? Or, for example, two. (For some time hesitates over the pack.) I can! I can afford it! I have willpower! Today I ate cottage cheese (God, disgusting, I hate cottage cheese!) And I have the right to eat cookies. (He opens the box and decisively swallows one quickly.) Hmm, I didn't feel the taste at all. Another...

Further scenarios may be different. Some of the fighters of the diet front will courageously put the box aside. Some will not stop until they finish it to the end. This does not mean that the former has a stronger will or more motivation; the decision to stop or not depends on what dietary phase you are in. When the suffering from the deprivation of delicious food reaches a high level, it becomes more difficult to resist. At the very beginning of the diet, this is easier to do. When deciding to go on a diet, sooner or later, you will visit both of these places more than once.

Chapter 3: The Third Principle - Eat When You Are Hungry, Understand Your Hunger Cues

Choosing an intuitive diet, we consciously abandon attempts to control the body. We take responsibility for the body and express our willingness to take care of it - just like an adult takes care of a child. We create a diverse, rich "nutrient medium" for the body, we give a choice and ... do not interfere.

Intuitive eating also means giving up trying to control your emotions with food. To control emotions, one has to master more mature psychic instruments. Not all of us are subject to total dietary thinking. Many people eat without dietary restrictions but get better because they use food to solve emotional problems. Many eat in various social situations, being unable to resist the sight and presence of food. And what kind of eater are you? What is your food scenario? Let's figure it out.

Cautious Eater

He is obsessed with healthy eating, as he imagines it. It does not mix proteins with carbohydrates, but carbohydrates with fats. Do not eat simple carbohydrates, GMOs, or eats only organic food. Practicing a raw food diet or vegetarianism. Shopping for a week is a half-day adventure, as the composition of each purchased product is studied with special care. A supermarket for a careful eater is about the same as a mined field for a sapper. Products on the shelves can poison his fragile body in minutes. Somewhere, among this liquid, loose, sweet, and spicy poisons, are hidden those very three or four names that are relatively safe. A cautious eater courageously makes his way among the hostile shelves in a desperate search for the edible.

Ready to go for food of the right quality to the other end of the city, get up at 6 in the morning to catch the farmers' market. Spends a lot of time planning the following meals.

Of course, there is nothing wrong with eating quality products and knowing what exactly gets on the table and in the refrigerator. The fundamental difference is in the amount of time and effort that such an eater spends thinking, searching for and buying the "right" food, as well as the genuine horror, disgust, and anger that cautious eaters are prompted to enter, for example, at McDonald's. A survival program is built into our brains from birth - so if we find ourselves in a situation where only food from McDonald's is available, most of us, with more or less pleasure and benefit, will nevertheless eat it - and survive. A cautious eater would rather starve than eat an "unhealthy" one.

Most of all, this type corresponds to the description of a new eating disorder - orthorexia (a painful desire for "proper" nutrition according to a special system).

"Professional Eater"

He is easy to identify - this is a person who is always on a diet. He is aware of all the new dietary innovations. He read the recently released book by a fashionable nutritionist. If you got a homework idea to find out how many kilocalories in a handful of ants - call him, he is in the know. These people determine the caloric content and fat content of products, barely glancing at them, accurately consider bread units. If a cautious eater thinks about food all the time, then a "professional" always thinks. He may not remember what he ate at dinner, but he perfectly knows how many calories his dinner "weighed."

Professional consumers, like cautious ones, completely cease to feel the taste and enjoyment of food. Many of them obsessively strive to lose weight and try laxatives or diet pills along the way; most of them are considering the possibility of bariatric surgery even in the presence of medical indications. Being a professional eater means walking the very fine line between trying to control what you eat and eating disorders.

Many professional eaters, despite the huge amount of knowledge on dietetics, systematically overeat. The reasons may be different - this is the "last time" before starting a new diet, which from tomorrow will deprive the professional eater of the opportunity to eat what he really wants, and reward himself with delicious food for a week of exemplary dietary behavior. As with careful eaters, contact with food causes them a lot of anxiety and stress. Food is perceived as an enemy, which must be subdued, defeated, and vigilantly controlled.

"Carefree Eater"

Consumers on the run, people eating and not breaking away from the work process, burying themselves on the TV screen, phone, computer - these are examples of careless eaters. A careless eater does not feel the taste of food, often does not even realize how much and what he just ate. Among the careless eaters, the following options can be distinguished:

– Chaotic. There is no time for a chaotic eater, or it is a pity to waste time on food. Therefore, he eats on the go, on the run, grabbing the first thing that comes to hand, eats without taste, stopping to eat, only when hunger really gnaws him from the inside. As a result, chaotic eaters often eat very illegibly and overeat.

– Failsafe. It is literally difficult for a trouble-free eater to resist eating, whether he is full or hungry. If food is nearby, he will eat, often without even realizing what he is eating. It is the trouble-free eaters - those same people who cannot pass by a vase of sweets without grabbing a handful from it and immediately putting everything they got out of their mouths.

– Member of the Clean Plate Society. This is a man whose mother and grandmother taught as a child that throwing away food is not allowed. The idea of leaving something on a plate causes him strong resistance, and the offer to simply throw out the rest is a holy horror. A member of the "Clean Plate Society" will be choking eating up at the restaurant because "it has already been paid for," and at home - because it is "wrong to throw it out." Often, such eaters eat up after children and partners and find ways to process even spoiled foods (you can cut mold from cheese and rub cheese into an omelet, boil acidifying soup, make crackers from drying bread).

– An emotional eater. Emotional eaters use food as a comforter, a means of mitigating negative emotions. They deal with sadness, boredom, anger, and frustration with a packet of chips or a few chocolates. The main problem of such consumers is that they do not have adequate tools to cope with negative emotions, and food is actually the only available means of processing.

Surely you recognize yourself in one of these types, and most likely not even in one. This is completely normal - our food style often includes several options for disturbed eating behavior.

Despite the fact that there are a lot of described types, in reality, there are only three variants of disturbed eating behavior: diet type, emotional, and external.

All the described food styles are various combinations of these three types of disorders. To exactly determine what violations are specific to you, we will use a questionnaire developed in 1987 by a Dutch psychologist, a leading specialist in the field of nutrition psychology. Answer questions quickly without hesitation - so you get an adequate result.

Possible answers: "never," "very rarely," "sometimes," "often," "very often." Choose the option that best suits your behavior in each of the situations described.

> If your weight begins to grow, do you try to eat less than usual?

> Do you try to eat less than you want at breakfast, lunch, dinner?

> Do you often refuse food or drinks because you are worried about your weight?

> Do you control the amount eaten?

> Do you choose food specifically to lose weight?

> If you overeat, will you eat less the next day?

> Do you try to eat less so as not to get better?

- How often do you try not to eat between meals, for the fact that you watch your weight?

- How often do you try not to eat in the evenings, for the fact that you watch your weight?

- Do you think about how much you weigh before you eat something?

- Do you have a desire to eat something when you are annoyed?

- Do you feel like eating something when you have nothing to do?

- Do you have a desire to eat something when you are depressed or upset?

- Do you have a desire to eat something when you are lonely?

- Do you feel like eating something when someone has let you down?

- Do you have a desire to eat something when something impedes the fulfillment of your plans?

- Do you feel like eating something when you anticipate that a nuisance will happen?

- Do you have a desire to eat something when you are alarmed, preoccupied, or tense?

- Do you have a desire to eat something when everything is wrong when everything falls out of your hands?

- Do you feel like eating something when you are scared?

- Do you have a desire to eat something when you are disappointed when your hopes are not fulfilled?

- Do you have a desire to eat something when you are excited or upset?

- Do you have a desire to eat something when you are tired or alarmed?

- Do you eat more than usual when the food is delicious?

- Do you eat more than usual when the food looks especially appetizing and smells?
- If you see delicious food, smell it, do you have an appetite?
- If you have something tasty, will you eat it immediately?
- If you pass by a pastry shop, whether you want to buy something tasty?
- If you pass by a café, would you want to buy something tasty?
- When you see how others eat, does it awaken your appetite?
- Can you stop when you eat something tasty?
- Do you eat more than usual while in a company (when others eat)?
- Do you try food when you cook?

Learn to Identify Your True Hunger Signals

Process the results of the questionnaire. For each "never," give yourself 1 point, "very rarely" - 2, "sometimes" - 3, "often" - 4 and "very often" - 5. In question 31, do the opposite (5 for "never" and 1 point for "very often"). Add up the points received for the first 10 questions and divide the amount by 10. Add up the points received for questions 11–23 and divide the amount by 13. Add up the points received for questions 24–33 and divide the amount by 10. You received 3 numbers that characterize your eating behavior.

Is It Craving or Hunger?

Restrictive (Dietary) eating behavior, the norm on this scale is 2.4. If your result is so much, a little less or a little more - you have no problems with food restrictions, you allow yourself to eat freely and at the same time eat reasonably enough.

If the result obtained exceeds the norm - most likely, you are a "cautious" or "professional" eater, your relationship with food is far from harmonious. You are afraid to eat, so as not to gain weight or guided by considerations of "usefulness."

If the result is much lower than normal - you eat uncontrollably, without restrictions, poorly aware of what and how you eat. Most often, a low result on this scale is combined with increases on two other scales and also means a violation of eating behavior.

Emotional eating behavior. The norm on this scale is 1.8. If the result you get is in line with the norm, you are not inclined to jam emotions. If the resulting figure is higher than normal - it is difficult for you to process emotions without resorting to food. The food in your life is not an enemy, but a comforter, psychotherapist, and friend. Most likely, your food style is an "emotional eater."

External eating behavior. The norm on this scale is 2.7. If your result is below the norm, you are not inclined to overeat in social situations or because the food is in plain sight and accessible. If you are above the norm, you are most likely a "trouble-free" eater who finds it difficult to stop when he starts eating. It is difficult to resist the sight of a delicious or simply lying meal. Such people usually believe that they should not have delicious food at home, since it will be eaten on the first day after purchase, and they eat significantly more at dinner with friends than alone.

Thus, a careful eater will have to first work on unconditional permission to eat, a careless one - on raising awareness, and a professional - on both characteristics of eating behavior.

Throw Away Those Weighing Scales

Now you know exactly what eating disorders are characteristic for you. The results are not a sentence, not a diagnosis, and they can be changed. In order to begin practical work, you will need:

1. A small notebook, notepad, file on the computer.

2. A phone with a camera or a small pocket camera.

3. Voice recorder (or a similar function in your smartphone).

4. Full-length mirror.

5. ... and a little courage.

Details on these in **Chapter 6**.

Believe the list is incomplete? It lacks willpower - a quality familiar to everyone who has ever dieted. The first few days you have it, and you are proud of it, then it disappears somewhere. In fact, to cope with your eating disorders, willpower is not needed. Neither is a weighing scale.

Forget about the power of will - it does not exist at all, according to the latest research by psychologists. You will need to understand and recognize the motives, most often the unconscious, that cause you to choose certain types of behavior over and over again. By understanding the motive, we can deal with unwanted behavior. And you have to find out that some people are much more prone to overeating due to genetic characteristics and education.

Chapter 4: The Fourth Principle - Be Present and Enjoy!

One day this can happen to any of us. You get on the scales, enter the value in the online calculator, or open the tables... Wow - obesity!

Let's talk about the most unpleasant, most abusive words of the three letters. No, they are not written on the fence. These are the words "weight" and "fat." Close your eyes for a minute: what associations do they cause you? Hardly anything good. We associate fat with folds on the body protruding underclothes, unhealthy, sloppy and unkempt, ugliness, and gluttony. "Weight" is a slightly more delicate name for the same phenomenon, but when we look at ourselves in a mirror all alone, we always call what we see "fat" and nothing else.

It's extremely rare to see full people on the covers of glossy magazines; moreover, on the covers, we see extreme harmony as if it symbolized beauty and health. Young women and men are universally preoccupied with the fight against fat in their own bodies (sometimes calling it "the fight against excess weight," but the target of the persecution is fat, and nothing else). It is often possible to hear the desire to "completely get rid of body fat" as if water and muscles are all that a healthy individual should consist of.

But is fat in itself bad? According to the famous American cardiologist Carl Lavie, a certified cardiologist at one of the largest cardiology centers in the United States, the fat in our body in the right amount (and this is probably more than you strive to have) is exactly what we need to live long and enjoy high-quality life. Completeness is understood exclusively incorrectly and described in a false way from many points of view. At the same time, the popularization of sports and intense physical training is unjustly overstated.

Studying unwanted folds in a mirror, we often think: and why do I need this fat, it would be better if it weren't at all! Bodybuilders strive to get rid of the slightest presence of fat in the body so that the muscles are even more beautiful, even more prominent - and we are used to considering such a body not only beautiful but also healthy.

In fact, fat performs a lot of useful functions in the body, and among the many of these functions, the following four are most important:

- Fat supports immunity. Cells that are "harbingers" of fat, called preadipocytes, work as special immune cells that neutralize dangerous bacteria and other microorganisms. This explains why dieters using the "drying" or detox method often start to get sick more often, experience pain, and experience various inflammatory processes.

- Glucose is stored in fat. In addition to muscles and liver, fat is the place where glucose is stored in the form of fat molecules. Studies of rats and humans with low body fat show chronically high glucose levels, just like diabetics do. This is because muscles that also store glucose as glycogen have limitations in the amount of glycogen they can contain. In diabetics, glucose does not enter the cells, because either they suffer from insulin deficiency (type 1 diabetes) or the cells do not respond to insulin. Without enough fat to store glucose for a rainy day, all free glucose can be in the blood. What does this mean? An exhausted, fat-free body can function just like a body with diabetes.

- Fat produces hormones. In addition to storing and releasing triglycerides, fat cells produce a huge number of hormones that are important for our health. Fluctuations in hormone levels can have a strong effect on the body. The hormone leptin is responsible for the feeling of fullness and signals to the body to stop and stop eating, and ghrelin - for the fact that hunger arose at a time when you have not eaten for a long time, and the body needs fuel. Insulin - our main anabolic hormone - controls the "energy stores" and their replenishment after each meal. Glucagon, adrenaline, and norepinephrine have the opposite effect of insulin, releasing fatty acids and glucose when they are needed. Fluctuations in the amount of fat mass can cause serious hormonal fluctuations and pose a threat to health.

- Fat metabolizes hormones. A large number of vital hormones are produced in fat cells. For example, in both men and women, testosterone in fat cells is converted to estrogen. That is why men with a large amount of fat mass acquire several feminine features - for example, breast enlargement (increase in estrogen), along with a decrease in libido (decrease in testosterone). The main stress hormone cortisol is also metabolized in fat cells. Cortisol has a poor reputation as a "stress hormone," however, it is vital for energy metabolism and is critical for survival. Cortisol in an inactive form is stored in subcutaneous fat.

Feel Your Body as You Eat

Put life aside "when I lose weight," "after I try this diet here." Remember that obesity is unique in that it is a disease exclusively human - in the wild, obesity does not occur.

It is widely believed that obesity is a dubious privilege of well-fed times, saying that in prehistoric times, there were no full people because you had to move more, and there is less. This is only partially true. Recall the images of the Paleolithic Venus, for example. Venus of Willendorf is a fat woman with a large belly and voluminous breasts. For sculptural images of Stone Age women, such extreme fullness was the norm. The term "obesity" itself officially appears in 1611, although the famous doctors of all time recognize their acquaintance with obesity, and often - in their negative attitude to it. So, the Indian doctor Sushruta, who lived in 800 BC., anticipating the achievements of modern plastic surgeons by making nasal reconstructions to their patients, associated obesity with diabetes and cardiovascular disease. After a few centuries, in 450 BC., Hippocrates will say: "Corpulence is not only a disease but also a warning to others."

Until the middle of the last century, fullness was the privilege of wealthy people, demonstrating a well-fed and happy life - and this fullness was never extreme. Wealthy people were what we now call "overweight" or "mildly obese" (BMI 25–30 or 30–35, respectively). Morbid obesity, in which BMI reaches 40 or more, is a modern phenomenon, previously unknown.

In a new way, the topic of excess weight in medicine sounded at the end of the XIX century. During this period, insurance companies began to search for factors affecting life expectancy, of course, in order to reduce costs. For the identified risk groups, it was planned to increase insurance payments or completely refuse to provide medical insurance. Weight could be easily measured and calculated - it is not surprising that the researchers turned to this. In 1869, the Belgian government set the task of developing a clear and simple criterion that allows you to estimate the number of obese people in a population quickly. The mathematician Adolphe Quetelet copes with this task, having invented the Body Mass Index - the ratio of body mass to the square of growth.

In 1897, the first "charts" appeared in the USA - tables of weight norms. The weight, which was recognized as a factor increasing the risk of mortality, was 20-30% higher than the average norm. The number of people in the population falling into these norms was extremely small. Being overweight was not in, and of itself considered a medical problem.

In the middle of the XX century, the situation is changing. Beauty standards, implying exceptional thinness, were approved in the 60s, and then, almost imperceptibly, being overweight - that is, any weight that does not meet these standards, is recognized not only as an aesthetic problem but also as a health problem. According to Susie Orbach, "The new epidemic of obesity is not just an increase in the number of such people, the reason for this is the revision of BMI in the direction of reducing the" criteria for obesity "in the last 6 years. If you look like Brad Pitt or George W. Bush, you are definitely overweight by now. If you are as dense as Russell Crowe, you are obese. As Paul Campos wrote in The Myth of Obesity, 38 million

Americans woke up in the morning and found themselves obese... Millions of dollars were invested by commercial weight loss programs in Shape up, America.

In fact, obesity turns out to be a man-made idea. Hence, you need to eat and be yourself. Be one with your food, and get rid of any ideas that served as a sales pitch for several big brands. Also, understand that the link between obesity and a number of dangerous diseases perfectly exploited the fear of death inherent in every person, and the vast market for diet programs, diet pills, and bariatric surgery began to develop more intensively than ever. You don't need to be in this "cage," do you?

What to Eat, When to Eat?

In the world of nightmares of a person who is overweight, in addition to the eternal, previously lost fight with sugar, usually, a lot of places are occupied by anxiety for one's health and fear of type 2 diabetes - one of the most typical. In fact, not only excess fat mass is a predictor of diabetes, but also a deficiency of fat in the body. In order to understand why this happens, it is important to understand what diabetes is and in what cases it occurs.

Insulin is one of the most important hormones produced by our body. It conducts the metabolic process, helping us translate the energy that we get from food into the cells of the body. The process by which our cells metabolize glucose molecules is completely unique. The fact is that our cells cannot simply capture glucose from the bloodstream. Imagine that a cell is a house whose doors are closed for glucose. Doors are closed, but energy is needed.

In order for a house-cell to open its doors and let glucose in, it needs the help of insulin. Insulin acts as a DHL courier, as a transporter, and is produced by the pancreas.
It is insulin that transfers glucose to muscles, fat, and liver cells, where it can be used as fuel. A healthy cell does not have any problems responding to insulin intake since, for this, they have many antennas on the roof of the house - cell receptors. However, if the couriers are constantly breaking in the door - the cells systematically survive the influx of large amounts of insulin as a result of the constant presence of glucose in the blood, which is typical when there is a large amount of refined sugar and simple carbohydrates in the food, then at some point the cells do not stand up ... And they start to adapt. They reduce the number of receptors - the owner of the house removes excess antennas. Chick truck, I'm in the house.

As a result, the house-cell with a reduced number of antennas becomes insulin resistant - it ceases to recognize the courier delivering glucose in the face and tells him: "Who are you? Bye Bye!"

What is the result? The owner of the house does not open the door to the bell of the courier who delivered glucose. He pretends that he is not at home, ignoring poor insulin, and leaving him to freeze at the doorstep. True, only the cell itself is worse from this - as a result, the delivered glucose does not enter it or does not receive enough.

The body, this wise and balanced system, is trying to find a quick solution to the problem. Which one? That's right, increase the amount of insulin, which the pancreas can cope with without problems. As a result, the body needs higher amounts of insulin to absorb the same amount of glucose.

This leads to the formation of a repeating cycle, which can lead to the development of type 2 diabetes. If you are already a type 2 diabetic, by definition, you have a lot of glucose in your blood. Misfit glucose flows through the bloodstream, instead of entering cells and being locked up in a store of spare energy. Freely staggering glucose is a poorly educated "fellow" with a knife and a crossbow, the longer it is in a free state in the body, the more harm it causes. The heart becomes a victim among other organs, the risk of stroke, cardiovascular disease, kidney disease, blindness increases.

What is important for us not to forget is that a chronic imbalance of blood sugar triggers this pathological cycle, independently on weight.

Insulin - our DHL courier - is not only involved in the delivery of glucose to cells. This is an anabolic hormone, and this means that it stimulates growth, promotes the formation of fat, promotes inflammatory processes, increases pressure, and increases the size of the heart muscle. When insulin levels are constantly high, it causes a disturbance in the secretion of other hormones. They can completely stop being produced or, conversely, start to stand out too quickly and intensively, which leads to unpredictable consequences. The body begins to function in extreme mode, and even if we manage to transfer it to normal operation, the natural ability of the body to restore its functions may be lost forever.

And this can happen with both a thin and a full man, absolutely regardless of his weight. And now, in fact, about the most interesting. Is it possible to eat consciously and intuitively while being insulin-resistant? Being a type 2 diabetic?

The answer is not only possible but also necessary. The life of a diabetic is constant monitoring, constant self-observation. Those who have self-observation skills live happily ever after. Therefore, in "diabetes management" in Western

European medicine (the management of a chronic disease is a stable medical term, which means, in essence, a system of procedures that allows you to maintain and improve the patient's normal quality of life, not to become disabled, and to avoid crises), today the main place it is nutritional awareness.

A study by Cara Miller et al. (2012) at Ohio University compared the standard diet choices program Smart Choices, based on the principles of dietary restrictions, and the Conscious Meals program (capital letters are used because this is a very specific program whose name is protected copyright) for diabetics. Since the main role in the life of a diabetic is not played by visits to the doctor, but by his own daily behavior, including eating, diabetics are standardly taught the techniques and skills of healthy eating, life, and disease management. Until recently, the nutrition of a diabetic was based on three basic principles:

1. This is impossible.
2. This is completely impossible.
3. But this is never possible.

The Smart Choices program is a well-known system for dividing products into "good," "so-so," and "terrible." Each group corresponds to the color of the traffic light - green, yellow, or red. Products from the green group (green vegetables) can be eaten without restrictions, products from the yellow one - with great care (carbohydrate-containing products are included there) and, finally, products from the red one - allow yourself as a big exception (this group includes any unbridled fast food and sweet soda).

The idea was that by following this nutrition plan, a diabetic would be able to maintain a stable weight and blood sugar. The problem, as usual, was that most diabetics could not survive this system without constant breakdowns, which is not surprising.

The study compared a group of diabetics following the Smart Choices system and a group of diabetics trained in Mental Nutrition and intuitive eating for people with diabetes. No statistically significant differences were found in changes in weight, BMI, and waist size. That is, people who ate everything that they wanted, found the same dynamics of weight as people following a restrictive diet with a predominance of vegetables and fruits. Both groups became less likely to eat as a result of training in nutritional skills, while the group that studied Conscious Nutrition consumed fewer sugars, ate foods with a lower glycemic load, and, as a result, the total amount of energy consumed was less (this coincides with my own observations, that intuitive and informed nutrition in itself leads to a significant reduction in sugar consumption - you just don't want sweets). It is worth noting that for patients with a dietary program, a change in eating style was characteristic immediately after training,

Thus, to answer the questions: what to eat, when to eat. I say anything, at any time. Your body, as the master of itself, will give you innate signals that provide you the best results in the long run.

This is what Marsha Handall, one of the Green Mountain at Fox Run Clinic staff, wrote back in the 70s.

- The number of peaks and drops in blood sugar levels decreases as you pay attention to how certain foods or eating behaviors affect blood sugar levels.
- By listening to yourself, you may find that your sensations after food that seemed desirable (cake, hamburger) are rather unpleasant. This reduces your cravings for junk food.
- You get more pleasure from eating, which ultimately leads to the fact that you eat less. To enjoy food, you need to choose exactly what you want at the moment, and be in this moment, be present consciously.
- You eat less because you are not deprived. The absence of food bans, the rule "eat whatever you want," leads to the fact that you stop eating because of guilt, a feeling of restriction, or protest ("let it go to hell, I want a cake!"). You only eat because you want some kind of food.

Thus, an intuitive lifestyle of eating is not only possible but also has a number of obvious advantages. Of course, the teaching of intuitive and informed nutrition for diabetics is carried out under the supervision of a nutritionist, endocrinologist, and taking into account the indications of a glucometer - but this is perhaps the only difference from an ordinary person.

Chapter 5: The Fifth Principle: Learning When Your Hunger Is Satisfied

Compulsive and paroxysmal overeating, are, of course, extremely unlucky eating disorders that have gotten along with anorexia, attractive in its mortal danger, and less gothic, but marked by a canopy of royal greatness bulimia.

How do I know if I am a compulsive eater or just love to eat? In essence, very simple. Compulsive eaters regularly turn to food in the absence of physiological hunger. This does not mean that the "normal" eater does not have any moments when the food is absorbed not because it is hungry, but because it looks appetizing or because it is a vacation, and "all-inclusive" is paid by your own money. However, unlike a compulsive eater, a normal eater recognizes discomfort signals - a feeling of heaviness in the stomach, drowsiness, heartburn - and calmly waits for the next moment of physiological hunger to eat. A compulsive eater, overeating, abusively curses himself, panics, goes into hysteria and despair, and ponders how to punish himself dietarily - sit down on Monday to a "brawl" then once again go to the gym, and so on. Since there can be several such moments in a compulsive eater during one day, this takes a huge amount of mental energy and leads to low self-esteem, depression, and chronic guilt.

The key point is not at all on how much you weigh; there are quite slender individuals among compulsive eaters. The key point is that the process of absorption of food has little to do with hunger. In fact, many compulsive eaters no longer know what hunger is.

There is a classic, widely cited study by Janet Polivy and Peter Herman of the University of Toronto, about how people on a restrictive diet lose their ability to feel hungry and recognize signs of satiety. In the study, the group of participants following the current diet and the group of people eating normally were tasked with comparing the different tastes of ice cream. All participants were divided into three subgroups. The first one was given two milkshakes to drink before offering ice cream for a test. The second was given to drink one milkshake before ice cream. The third was given nothing at all but ice cream. Next, the participants were offered three different varieties of ice cream, asked to rate them by eating as much as they wanted.

As a result, in the group of people eating normally, the maximum amount of ice cream was consumed by a subgroup to which not a single milkshake had crossed. Those who drank one ate less ice cream. Those who drank two are much less.

And on dieters, the opposite results were obtained. Those who did not get a single cocktail ate the least ice cream. Those who drank one cocktail ate more, but those who drank two ate most. Researchers called the phenomenon discovered "dis-inhibition" - anti-suppression, that is, the process opposite to the usual dietary suppression of the normal nutrition process. "I have already violated the diet anyway, so you can tear yourself away until I return to it again."

Dieting and bouts of gluttony, excessive physical activity in the gym, and attempts to skip the next meal, absorbing much less or much more food than your body needs - all these are disturbing types of food eating patterns. They do not necessarily reach the level of eating disorders, but necessarily invade a person's life, disorganizing and destroying it. Most experts on violated types of nutrition come to the conclusion that sooner or later, any diet leads to a breakdown and subsequent attack of gluttony, resulting in a closed cycle "diet-overeating."

Negative thoughts and beliefs trigger dietary behavior. We already spoke about them earlier, as a characteristic feature of a person with an upset diet. No diet begins with the fact that a person looks at himself in the mirror and thinks: "I look great! But can I go on a diet? "Any diet begins with the experience: "I am fat, my stomach is bulging, my hips are too wide, and fat is hanging on my hands ..." Any diet starts with negative thoughts. People who hang in repeated long-term dietary cycles suffer from what they call "bad body thoughts," a negative attitude toward their own bodies.

The modern cultural climate is an ideal environment for cultivating a negative image of one's own body. The average model has a 13 to 19% weight deficit according to medical standards. With 15% weight deficiency, anorexia nervosa is diagnosed. Of course, there are metabolically thin people who, without effort and even against desire, fall into this category. According to statistics, there are about 3-5% of them in the population. Glossy literature offers everyone else to work - with the help of a diet and a gym - to reach this level, hinting that with a "proper" diet and continuous plowing in the gym, it is possible. So, this is not true. In addition to the direct destructive effect on the image of oneself, these cultural standards also have an indirect. As I already wrote, there is no diet without breakdowns. During a breakdown, the diet victim hates himself and thinks: how did it happen - after all, others succeed (according to legends), but I never have! This is a direct route to diet pills and bariatric surgery (stomach volume restriction surgery). So a woman, not being able to take her own image, does plastic surgery, because she does not believe that she can be attractive without changing.

In addition to negative thoughts about the body, dietary behavior also forms negative thoughts about "bad" or "bad" food. Today it has already become commonplace: any student will teach you, like our father, that bad food is a hamburger and French fries, and good food is a salad leaf and an apple. We have become terribly educated in this part, and this has its drawbacks.

Each diet-overeating cycle begins with the main thing: a sense of control. This time I will succeed, we tell ourselves, armed with a book of a new diet guru, scales, and a refrigerator with chicken breast and celery. At the initial stage, the dieter feels like a hero, refusing the usual tasty things, small carbohydrate feasts at work, and "coffee" with friends, implying a sample of all the cakes on the menu. A sense of control and "false" hope are the two main feelings with which any diet begins. And this, I tell you, is enough to feel better. And when the scales show the first "minus" - self-esteem rises, and life begins to play with bright colors.

When Are You Really Full?

It would seem that everything is simple - not Newton's binomial. To normalize weight, you need to normalize the relationship with food. In order to normalize the relationship with food, you need, in fact, three important things - to find out and understand how I eat and what I'm eating, to understand what is happening to my body image (people globally dissatisfied with how they look are not extra pounds on the abdomen or hips, but by itself as a whole, are much more inclined to "break off" and periodically gain kilograms - in retaliation for their own bodies because they are so unattractive) and allow them to control the choice of food, time and volume of the body eaten, that is, hunger.

If not hunger regulates meals, then what? Emotional state - time. I eat because I feel sad, lonely or angry, I eat as a reward for the work done, or vice versa, so that I can postpone the start of a business that is unpleasant for me, finally I eat because I'm overworked, take responsibility, and I can't revise the schedule, and I need insulin bursts of energy to move on. We also examined these reasons earlier.

What else regulates your meals? In situations where hunger does not manage food, everything is in charge.

- I eat "for the company." My husband came from work, and the children came from school, I am not hungry, but I eat, because this is a way of communication or a means of structuring this communication.

– I eat because the social situation is pushing me to do this. I came to visit, and it is inconvenient to refuse. Guests came to me, and not to feed them - inhospitable.

– I eat because food is in front of my nose, and since it lies here, I'll eat it (something that almost all compulsive eaters say - if it's not good for me to eat, I can't have this in the house).

– I eat because I'm used to certain actions in my life being accompanied by food. Saturday's grocery shopping trip, a trip to the cinema with children, and much more put us in the face of many cultural catering enterprises that open their doors to us so tempting - you cannot cook, don't clean the dishes, and we're already here anyway...

– I eat because I am thirsty, and I am not used to distinguishing thirst from hunger. I eat because I am cold, I eat because I have a headache, every signal from the side of the body that is not hunger, and I interpret as hunger, because I am too anxious or too difficult to accept hunger as it is.

– I eat, "so as not to spoil" and "well, do not throw it away," that is, I use the body as a trash bin.

– I eat from fatigue, because I cannot afford to rest, and instead "spur" myself food. I eat to be left alone - because this is the only way to stay in silence. I eat so as not to start a business that I do not want to start.

And what kind of feelings does the feeling of hunger make you feel when you still experience it? Observe yourself. It is very important to understand. When you do, you will know when it is your obsession that is pushing you to eat more food further.

Hunger Scale

A very necessary skill when losing weight and following an intuitive diet is to learn to distinguish between physical and emotional sensations associated with food. Why is it important to "recognize" hunger? How to control the appetite for losing weight? How does overeating occur? Here are tips for you.

Hunger and Appetite

"Hunger" and "appetite" - these two concepts are often confused, so for a start, we will deal with terminology. Hunger refers to the physiological sensation of a need for food that occurs when enough time has passed after a meal, and the body needs a new portion of nutrients.

Appetite (or psychological, emotional hunger), we will call the desire to eat when, from the point of view of physiology, a person is full. Suppose you saw something very tasty in a store window and immediately decided that you should definitely try this dish. Or something happened, and you hurry to "seize" the troubles that have fallen on you. Or you cannot deny yourself the pleasure after a hearty lunch to drink tea with a cake with colleagues. There are a great many such situations, so it is very important to learn to distinguish between physiological and psychological hunger.

What are their main differences? Physiological hunger occurs gradually, while appetite occurs suddenly. The physiological hunger is patient, he can wait a bit until the opportunity to eat, but his psychological "brother" requires immediate satisfaction. Moreover, a person becomes physically ill if, at that moment, he does not eat the desired piece of cake or a dish he likes.

Physiological hunger can be satisfied with any meal, even a piece of bread, in contrast to psychological hunger, when, as a rule, you want either a specific meal (for example, lamb chops) or a certain group of products (say, something sweet).

Hunger is manifested by physical sensations - a feeling of emptiness in the stomach, sucking under the spoon. If it is not satisfied for a long time, symptoms such as dizziness, trembling hands, and nausea may appear. Emotional symptoms are also connected to them - irritation, anger, aggression. Appetite does not live in the stomach, but in the head and manifests itself as thoughts about food. Moreover, if a person eats a prohibited product, then very often after that, he has a feeling of guilt or lack of satisfaction from the eaten piece, which was expected.

To understand the differences in hunger and appetite and remember about them, the following hunger scale table will also help you.

Psychological hunger (appetite)	Physical hunger
Comes suddenly.	Comes gradually.
It manifests itself as a craving for specific food (I want to get a taste).	It is characterized by openness to various products or dishes.
Lives in the head (thoughts about food appear).	Lives in the stomach (there is a feeling of emptiness in the stomach, "sucks under the stomach").
Requires immediate, immediate satisfaction.	Patient.
It is paired with emotion (positive or negative).	Arises from physical need (if more than two hours have passed since the last meal).
Associated with mindless, automatic ingestion of food.	Associated with the deliberate choice and awareness of the food process.
It doesn't pass even if the stomach is already full.	Passes when hunger is already satisfied.
Often generates a feeling of shame for food eaten.	Food is positioned as a necessity.

After you learn to distinguish between hunger and appetite, you will need to do the following each time they appear. If it's hunger, evaluate it on a scale from 0 to 4 (how this is done, I will tell you a little later), and if it's appetite, ask yourself two questions: "What exactly made me want to eat this product?" and "In what other way can I satisfy this need?" When you come up with a way, be sure to put this idea into practice.

If you can't find a solution, then watch others and try to find out how they do it. Or turn on your imagination and imagine how the person you admire behaves in such a situation. Perhaps you can find a way out by answering a question like: "How would my intuitive eater coach act in my place?" And of course, if you have done all of the above, but could not find the answer, indulge yourself. It will only get better as time passes.

Drawing your hunger Scale

Now make a scale of your own manifestations of hunger. To do this, take a sheet of A4 paper and put the numbers from 0 to 4 on it so that they occupy the entire left column. After that, opposite each figure, you need to describe:

- physical sensations that you experience at this stage of hunger;
- emotions that you feel at this moment;
- thoughts that you have;

- Your usual behavior in such a situation.

What Sensations May Correspond to the Points on This Scale?

The easiest way to start the description is with the numbers 0 or 4. "Four" - this is the most intense feeling of hunger that you ever experienced when you were ready, as they say, to eat an elephant. The description of the "four" may look something like this:

- physical sensations: a very strong feeling of discomfort (or even pain) in the stomach, nausea, dizziness, trembling hands;
- emotions: irritation, anger, aggression;
- thoughts: run to the nearest grocery store or shawarma stand;
- Behavior: eagerly absorb the first food that catches your eye, if food is not available, break down on others.

After the Quartet, I recommend describing "Zero." This figure corresponds to a state of pleasant satiety after eating (but not overeating!). I warn you right away: difficulties can arise with a description of physical sensations. As a rule, we feel good signs of hunger or, conversely, overeating. But how to describe the manifestations of satiety? Listen carefully to yourself. This may be a feeling of fullness or pleasant warmth in the stomach. It may be helpful to note which symptoms are absent.

It is easier with an emotional state: usually, its calmness, relaxation. But drowsiness, as a rule, does not happen. If it is, be careful: perhaps you have already described the symptom of overeating. As for thoughts, at this moment, they are extremely rarely associated with food. Finally, the last and in this case, a very important point is behavior: what are you doing at this moment and how much time after satiety can you do without food?

After you have described the extreme points of the scale, go to either "one" or "three." As practice shows, the greatest difficulties arise when describing hunger for a "deuce" - such an intermediate feeling that overweight people very often miss.

How to Avoid Overeating?

The task, frankly, is not easy, because in ordinary life, we do not differentiate this condition, but it is very important because, in the future, it will allow us to control the feeling of hunger. After you follow it and you will clearly know your criteria, the main task will be to provide yourself with food when the feeling of hunger corresponds to the number "2".

There is one pitfall that you need to learn how to get around. When a person is very busy or keen on something, he does not listen to his physical sensations. It can be an interesting work or a solution to some complex problem when we are immersed in a very pleasant trance state - the state of the so-called flow. At this moment, we are fully focused on our lesson and as active as possible, but at the same time, absolutely disconnected from our body. This condition is familiar to many - people in creative professions, women who enjoy, for example, sewing or knitting, parents who are passionately playing with children.

Being in a state of flow, we may simply not notice the emerging feeling of hunger. Therefore, you need to come up with a way to remind yourself that it's time to pause and take care of your body. Because it is so important? Yes, because in a state of flow, a person loses track of time and can do what he loves for many hours in a row. When he finally stops, it is then that all the sensations of a starving body will flood over, and at the same time, the emotions associated with them.

Needless to say, the feeling of hunger at this moment will be maximum. Overeating in such a situation is simply inevitable!

Chapter 6: The Sixth Principle: Burn You're "Never Ever" List

According to statistics, 95% of any diets result in a person gaining exactly the same number of kilograms, often more. Why?

1. Genetics

Our bodies are not so much "sculpted" from the outside, like a new fitness program advertisement trying to show. About 40 to 70% of our body weight is genetically determined. This means that outside intervention can help manage about 30-50% of the weight; the rest will surely be gained again.

2. Evolution

Evolutionary fat cells played a large role in the process of reproduction and survival of mankind. As a result, our body has the ability to accumulate fat cells after each short period of fasting. This is especially true for girls of puberty. To prepare the female body for reproduction, the body produces fat cells and lays them in the chest, on the hips, stomach of the girl. The limiting diet in this period leads to the fact that the hyper-production of fat cells begins. In addition, the overproduction of lipogenic enzymes (helping to accumulate fat substances) begins. As a result, as soon as the girl stops the diet and begins to eat normally, her body starts the work of fat factories with doubled power and speed. So every calorie consumed is instantly carefully converted into fat.

3. Adaptation

The body tends to adapt to the current model of energy consumption. Each body, of course, has its own optimal functioning point, within which it receives the optimal amount of food at those moments when the owner of this body is really hungry, stops consumption at the time of saturation, and daily performs some kind of physical activity.

If the body receives too much "fuel," the metabolism "accelerates," the body begins to function more intensively. If less fuel starts to flow, the body has to deal with it, limiting, slowing down the metabolism. During the period from 24 to 48 hours from the start of the restrictive diet, the level of metabolism in humans decreases from 15 to 30%.

It is well known that, in coping with the onset of the "hungry" period, the body burns not so much fat as muscle tissue to compensate. However, the more muscle, the higher the metabolism, the more "fuel" burns!

Hence, you should delete the never foods from your list. While you keep punishing yourself, your body is adapting to being just you in its own way(s)! Also, as noted previously, having certain foods on your never-ever list and you can't have them, you're going to end up feeling deprived. This, as also noted, is the onset of eating disorders that prove more a difficult puzzle to solve.

My Food Rules

Intuitive nutrition is becoming popular, which is not surprising - we are increasingly faced with the unpleasant consequences of the desire to make the diet "healthy." Typically, the diet alternates with eating disorders, followed by punishment with guilt and new attempts to eat properly. How does intuitive nutrition help?

Having begun to look for an alternative, many come across ideas that are called "intuitive nutrition," and this is wonderful - it's only a pity that in the information space, these words are called many things that are not related to it. To make it a lot easier, let us consider the "food rules" and bust myths about intuitive eating and intuitive eaters.

Myth # 1: Intuitive Nutrition Is Chaos and Permissiveness.

You often hear: "I tried. I bought myself a cake, chips, donuts... For two months, I ate what I wanted, recovered by 7 kg! Thank you, I don't want to. "Indeed, such a diet implies the ability to eat anything - including donuts, but relying on the signals of one's own body about hunger and satiety, and not solving one's own emotional problems with food. Not having mastered these basic skills, it's too early to buy cakes.

Myth # 2: It's the Choice Between Buckwheat and Oatmeal for Breakfast.

The opposite myth, especially characteristic of "amateur consultants" - people without special education, who have mastered their own weight loss and sell their services to others. For this mythology, the concept of abandoning dietary thinking is incomprehensible, and they describe intuitive nutrition as the possibility of choosing allowed foods in a narrow "corridor," most often low-calorie, low-carb, or with a low glycemic index. Such nutrition is no different from a normal diet and does not lead to a solution to problems.

Awareness - inclusion, and enjoyment of the process. Unfortunately, diet corporations are promoting a completely different approach.

Very often, this type of diet is called "conscious" nutrition because awareness is similar to the "consciousness" instilled in us from childhood. And now it seems to us that "conscious nutrition" is conscious. "I won't choose a cake. I'll choose low-fat cottage cheese."

This approach has no relation to conscious or intuitive nutrition. This is another dietary trap that has only two equally unpleasant outcomes: a food breakdown or an obsession with the topic of "proper" nutrition.

Awareness - presence in the present moment, inclusion, and enjoyment of the process. Unfortunately, diet corporations are promoting a completely different approach.

Myth # 3: This Is a "Flexible Control," You Can Eat Anything, but Limiting Portions/Calories

Eat whatever you like. Eat anything. But in portions no more than a glass, every two hours. Nutritionists are well aware that diets do not work. But how to solve the problem of weight loss without restrictions?

The idea of "flexible control" is becoming more and more popular - individual restrictions disguised as "free food." Studies show that people who do nothing with their diet show a lower BMI over a longer period of time than those who use "flexible controls."

Food Diary "in a New Way"

In fact, we were all born as intuitive eaters. The baby is worried, turns his head, looking for his mother's chest, and cries until he gets food. He does this only when he is hungry. A well-fed baby stops eating and does not start until it is hungry.

Children who are allowed in the family to maintain this natural eating style for them, independently regulate the amount of energy entering the body. Sometimes they eat a lot, pleasing their parents with a good appetite, even sometimes when they need a very small amount of food.

Growing up, children, like babies, are able to regulate the intake of the necessary substances, relying on the internal signals of hunger and satiety. You just need to give them that opportunity.

Intuitive Nutrition: Where to Start?

Where to start the organization of intuitive nutrition in the family? Take the following into consideration:

1. All Products Are Equal, All Bodies Are Good

We agree with family members, including children, that we no longer divide food into "harmful" and "healthy," "healthy" and "unhealthy," and "good" and "bad." And exactly the same thing we do with our body: we will no longer evaluate ourselves and other people according to their size.

Why? Because it destroys our positive attitude towards our own bodies and forms the understanding in the minds of children that "fat" is equal to "bad." Stupid, ugly, unlucky, angry - all this is fat.

In the life of a child, there are quite a few chances to suddenly gain weight and experience the horror that now it is his turn to be judged, ridiculed, and unloved. Most children, imperceptibly and effortlessly reduce weight gain when they begin to grow.

Getting rid of fatphobia - the fear of becoming "fat" and hostility to the owners of large bodies - is much more difficult.

2. Down with Dietary Thinking

We believe that we can control how our children will eat and how their bodies will develop. This is actually a utopian fantasy. Children have an inborn appetite and interest in food. How the child will eat - a lot or a little, with interest or absent-mindedly, whether he will love broccoli or prefer sweets, and which body - large, with a large fat mass, thin, with a minimum of muscle and fat, or dense and muscular - he will form - largely predetermined genetically and microbiologically.

All we can do is give the child a role model of healthy, normal nutrition.

We, parents, can try to influence this by regulating the nutrition and the amount of movement of the child, but the result of our impacts will be minimal, the efforts will be huge, and most importantly, the child will receive probable mental injuries.

We don't know which genetic cards are "dealt" to our children until they are "played out" - and this will happen in adolescence. All we can do is give the child a role model of a healthy, normal diet.

3. We Agree on the Shore

Children begin to eat poorly when their parents cannot agree on how to feed them. If you decide to turn on an intuitive track, try to enlist the support of your partner. Print articles about research that show that intuitive nutritionists maintain a lower and more stable BMI throughout their lives. And most importantly, introduce him to the data that children who are put on a diet are highly likely to develop eating disorders and gain weight in the future.

4. Get Rid of Our Own "Cockroaches"

It is impossible to organize meals without starting from yourself. Reading my book – The Flow of Intuitive Eating, which you are, you find out for yourself what beliefs about weight and nutrition exist in your head and how this relates to personal history.

In your family, it was impossible to leave food on a plate? Was it a sin to throw away food? Or, perhaps, you have grown up in the belief that you need to limit yourself and that any "tasty" food will certainly manifest itself during weighing? Have you been forced to eat something that you don't like, have you been taught to "eat everything in a row," "not to sort out"? These educational strategies will certainly affect the way you eat and how you feed your children.

5. Making Food a Shared Responsibility

We all, even children, are equally responsible for our food. Put a shopping sheet, a pencil on a twine in the kitchen, and ask all family members to mark what they wanted to eat during the week, but there weren't such products at home. Ask the children who are not able to write about what products they would like to see at home. Make stocks of these products without being afraid that chocolate, ice cream, croissants, or halva will be on the list.

6. "Are You Hungry?" Is the First Step, the Most Important Question?

For each request for food from the child, ask him if he wants to eat. "May I have some candy?" - "Do you want to eat?" "When will we have dinner?" - "Are you hungry?" "Will I make myself a sandwich?" "Are you hungry?"

Access to food is possible only with a positive answer to this question. If it seems to you that the child is not hungry, but specifically says that he is hungry in order to get the desired treat, then most likely it is. When transferring children to intuitive nutrition, a period follows when the children "check" whether access to their beloved and desired food is really maintained.

Older children often try first to find out what kind of food we plan to offer them. "What have we got for dinner?" They ask. And if you tell them that cabbage schnitzels are for dinner, you will suddenly find that they are not at all hungry and very disappointed. However, it is worth noting that you joked and actually said you were having pizza for dinner, the same children in a flash turn into very hungry.

Do not get fooled by this. Let your question, "Do you want to eat?" always be the answer to the question, "What do we have for dinner?"

7. "What Exactly Do You Want?" - The Second Step

If the answer to the first question is yes, ask the child what exactly he wants. No, you don't have to stand at the stove all day and cook for the children everything they wish. Your duty is to find out what their food and taste preferences are at the moment, and if such food is not at home, note that it would be worth buying.

Children are very flexible creatures, and at the same time, they very clearly know what they want. True, they do not yet know how to discover this knowledge in themselves. Do not make a decision for the child, even if he is confused and cannot understand what he wants. Show him that finding the best combination of foods or dishes for his current hunger is a game with a detective bias.

"Do you want hot or cold?" - Even this simple question greatly narrows the search. "Do you want meat, bread, vegetables, or fruits?" "Do you want to have eggs in this dish?" "Could it be porridge?" "Is it soft, hard, crunchy, thin?"

Children enthusiastically begin to play the food "guessing game" because, for them, this means that at the moment, the attention of the parents belongs completely to them. Explain to the children that a positive answer to the question means that they presented themselves as having already eaten the selected dish and experienced a feeling of "coincidence" of the sensations and requests received.

8. "Have You Eaten Up?" - The Third Step

As soon as a child loses interest in food, is distracted, takes too long a pause, begins to play, or chat with other children - again, it is time to clarify what is happening. "Have you eaten up?" You ask the child, and this means that you are mentally prepared to let him go from the table and give you the opportunity to return to the game, pack the unfinished food wrap, and put it in the refrigerator.

It is unacceptable to try to regulate the amount eaten by a child, whether in the direction of increasing or decreasing.

The same thing must be done if the child has eaten everything to the end, but continues to remain at the table. Perhaps for the sake of communication, but maybe he has experience when he was already refused the second portion, and he does not dare to ask for more?

As said, it is unacceptable to try to regulate the amount eaten by a child, whether in the direction of increase or decrease. Remember: any of your attempts to resort to coercion in relation to eating in one direction or another will certainly meet with powerful resistance.

9. Legalization of Prohibited Products

One of the hottest topics is children and sweets. Most kids love sweets. Sweets are food that gives instant energy, which is very much appreciated by active children. They symbolize the summer holidays and free time with friends, holidays, gifts - all that children love so much!

There are no children equally committed to any sweets; each child has a preference. Find them out. It can be kinder surprises, chips, marmalade bears, or lollipops - whatever it is; it will be food that you do not approve of.

Tell the child that from now on, he will be able to decide how much his favorite food he wants to eat and when. Buy as many packs as the child can eat for 10-12 times - the prohibited product must be intentionally in excess. Give your child open access to this product and come to terms with the fact that for several days, he will eat only this.

No child chooses sweets as his main meal as part of his free eating style.

Replenish the supply of the product as soon as it is half-empty - the child must constantly receive confirmation that the marmalade bears will not run out. In the range from several days to several weeks, you will see how the child's interest in this product will fade away.

Of course, a new treat will appear. Do the same with this. No child in the framework of a freestyle of food chooses sweets as the main food. Children choose cheese, chicken, sandwiches, pasta, cucumbers, bananas, soup, zucchini, broccoli, and semolina - even in those families where the parents have the most terrible childhood memories of these products.

10. Personal Shelf

Give each minor family member a personal grocery shelf. It can be a vegetable basket in the refrigerator, or it can be a drawer in the kitchen dresser. Help the child in acquiring his favorite, at the moment, delicacies, not limiting or commenting on his choice. Explain to all family members that this is an "untouchable reserve" that belongs only to that family member and no one else.

Regularly replenish stocks as soon as less than half is left. If necessary, hang a nameplate on the shelf. Such a shelf is a guarantee of a child's peaceful relationship with sugar-containing products and the basis that when he gets out of parental control, he will not overeat sweets daily.

Experience with obese people, whose childhood was in the 60-70s in Western Europe, showed that the strategy of categorically restricting sweets, popular in those years, has very dire consequences.

Many of these patients reported that they began to gain catastrophic weight, being beyond parental control. Being by that time completely independent people in all other areas, in nutritional terms, they remained children, longing for a convenient moment to finally get hold of sweets and eat them to the dump.

Most mistakes in children's nutrition are based on an unconscious belief that we can teach them to eat one way or another, prompting them to this or forbidding them something. In fact, children are born into the world already able to eat and develop immediate, individual nutritional preferences during the first years of life. Our task as parents is to support them, to give them a choice.

Intuitive nutrition is a model that allows a child to raise responsibility for how he nourishes himself and to reduce parental anxiety based on the idea that we can make our children's bodies - or our own - be different from what nature bequeathed to them.

Why Does It Work?

The problem of overeating is only partially related to food. It is important not only what we eat, but how and why we do it. Every emotion - anger, boredom, fear, anxiety - has its own cause. None of the problems can be solved simply by having lunch. Food can only comfort and distract for a short while. As a result, you still have to deal with the source of anxiety, but by that time, you will build up extra pounds. Having a free will allows you to express yourself more and let nature play out your diets, dietary requirements for an ultimately better you!

Intuitive Activities

In any case, you should also prefer to choose different types of activity. As for physical activity, the same rule applies as for food: you decide how much and what to do. You can go to the fitness club, run, swim, waltz or just walk in the park - the main thing is to give pleasure. When at least once you feel a boost of energy after class, you can determine what is best: a couple of minutes in the morning to lie in bed or do morning exercises.

An American doctor who lost more than 20 kg of excess weight after having learned about intuitive eating and exercise, called the above principles nutrition of common sense. "It's funny," he said, "but if we give up the rules and restrictions and learn to eat intuitively in accordance with the signals of our body, it will practically not differ from the generally accepted norms of healthy eating.

See? You are a step closer!

Chapter 7: The Seventh Principle - Forget the Concept of 3 Meals a Day

Breakfast lunch dinner? 1200 calories and 2 snacks? One diet-free day a week? Forget it.

At first, you can experience hunger 5, 6, 8 times a day! There is nothing wrong with this, and it will not lead to weight gain - remember the fractional nutrition system, in which people eat 5-7 times a day and lose weight. Eat calmly 8 times a day, if there is such a need, trying to obey the main commandment - to start eating in a state of tangible, but not extreme hunger and stop in a state of "a little full, he'll enter again."

At this stage of the nutrition setting, it is important that at any time when you feel hungry, you can have a variety of foods. Extremely often, customers, inspired by the idea of adjusting their nutrition, agree to wait until the physiological hunger comes but do not care about the availability of food. As a result, a person experiences an extremely uncomfortable state: I know for sure what I want to eat, but... nothing!

Its consequence is the appearance of "preventive feeding," that is, a situation where I eat without being hungry in order to prevent a feeling of hunger. In this situation, it helps to think of oneself as a very small child, an infant. What do we do if we need to leave a child for a while? Are we leaving the babysitter expressed milk or a mixture? Spread apples, dried and cottage cheese pancakes on a shelf? No one expects a child to wait patiently when he is fed: the child will receive food when he is hungry. You too.

At this stage, any person mastering the science of nutrition settings has a lot of practical questions. What to do, because at work there is a break at a certain hour? What to do, because we decided to eat everything together?

To make food available in the workplace, you need to bring it there. The same applies to mother sitting at home with her children: after waking up all day, she may find that there is only "children's" food that she doesn't want to eat, but hasn't found tasty and nutritious food for her in the house. That is why it is very useful to keep a couple of units of food cooked and frozen for you in the refrigerator at work - for example, a container with your favorite soup or vegetable stew with chicken.

Arrange at home that since you are reconfiguring your entire body, you will not necessarily participate in family lunches or dinners. If you are not hungry, you do not have to sit at the table with everyone and choke on food - set aside food for a while. Practice shows that this time comes pretty quickly - from 15 minutes to half an hour.

Our entire food history, both phylogenetic, that is, historical, and ontogenetic, that is, individual, which everyone has personally, makes us forget how to listen and ask the body when and what he wants. Eat while they give! If you don't reach, you won't leave the table! For mom, for dad, aunt, and uncle! All this experience teaches us NOT to listen to what we really need, and therefore we find ourselves where we find ourselves - quarreling with the body, making food, body fuel, and a means of obtaining pleasure and energy, a black demon tempting the poor us, an enemy.

I am categorically opposed to "stop eating and going to the gym." Have mercy on yourself. Rushing to engage in a gym without preparation, you inflict a lot of micro-traumas on your body that cannot be prevented. For people with increased body weight, you need either special medical fitness on special equipment, under the guidance of a specially trained physiotherapist to work with obesity, or the most non-traumatic, gentle types of physical activity - Nordic walking (stick support unloads vulnerable joints), swimming (water absorbs loads and supports the whole body). Of course, I am aware that people whose ancestors built communism for several generations in a row are prone to masochism in the name of a lofty idea, but there is a limit to everything. In addition, overcoming constant pain greatly reduces motivation, and, as we already understood, physical activity is necessary to maintain metabolism.

Each diet period (probably sticking to the three meals a day mantra) slowing down the metabolism, ends with the fact that the victim of the diet absorbs even more fat, experiences atrocious attacks of appetite and accumulates a greater percentage of fat in relation to body weight.

The fact that dietary behavior is catastrophically destructive for the human body and personality did not become known yesterday. One of the key research on this topic was done back in 1944 at the University of Minnesota. The goal was to study the effects of a "half-starved" existence. A group of healthy men, physically and mentally, was put on a 6-month diet, extremely carefully balanced in terms of vitamins, minerals, and protein, but containing about 50% of calories from the usual level of consumption of the subject. Men consumed approximately 1,570 calories per day (this is far from the limit - low-carb crash diets can contain no more than 600–1000 kcal!). The nutritional scheme almost completely coincided with the popular and fashionable diets. By the time the male participants lost about 25% of their initial weight, Researchers had noted significant personality changes. Participants became depressed, constantly sleepy, irritable, and lethargic and had difficulty concentrating. In addition, their food turned into an obsession. They spoke almost nothing but food, cooking methods, delicacies, weight loss, and hunger. After that, to say that grunts and sudden bouts of crying "diet" are associated with a deficiency of magnesium and B vitamins - more than frivolous.

In the second part of the experiment, participants were allowed to eat whatever they wanted. The victims of the experiment regularly overate to such an extent that they became ill and needed medical intervention, experienced intense hunger, and quickly gained weight due to fat mass. Many lost the muscularity characteristic of them before the experiment, and some gained more weight than the initial.

Only after the weight has completely returned to the initial level, the process of stabilization of the energy and emotional level of the participants began.

You Have the Right to Eat

Imagine that you have waited - you really feel a real feeling of hunger. Great news! What do you do if you are really hungry? Eat!

Until now, you often scolded yourself for what you want to eat, and experienced feelings of guilt and panic in connection with hunger. From this very moment, hunger is your friend and helper, your guide to body contact. When you experienced hunger, you restrained it, getting a feeling of greater control as a result, and subsequently coped with the experienced deprivation through attacks of gluttony. From now on, your feeling of hunger gives you the right to eat, and exactly what you want, the moment you want. No need to wait for the treasured hour in the schedule, no need to suffer and nibble yourself, that you want a steak, not celery. This is the only way to take responsibility for the functioning of your body. Everything else is on auto-pilot and will regulate itself. Stop worrying!

Chapter 8: The Eight Principle - How to Practice Mindfulness Eating and Shut down Negative Thoughts

The initial phase of "tuning" your own body for his own needs is usually not easy. "All of this is wonderful, doctor, but how is this to be implemented? I have work. I have children who need to be taken to classes, and I have absolutely no time to think about it! " To facilitate the process, I tried to formulate the most important rules. Usually, they write - rational nutrition, as if irrational - this is bad. And we will eat irrationally - as the body needs, but not the brain - and then it will answer us with gratitude, health, and harmony.

Another fundamental principle of intuitive nutrition: a varied food should be constantly available, should be nearby, at arm's length. Always. Compulsive eaters often have extremely little food at home, as they either diet or almost nothing can be eaten, or they are afraid of an overeating attack - and then it is better not to keep "dangerous" food at home. For an intuitive eater, it is important to have access to the widest possible variety of products so that at the right time, you can make the best choice that is in harmony with the needs of the body. Why is it important? Because having found the optimal combination at the moment, you will be satisfied with the minimum amount of food necessary for the current energy level of the body.

At home, at work, wherever there is an opportunity to make food supplies - make them. When you are hungry, you should have the maximum possible choice. What if hunger catches on the road or where food cannot be stored? Carry it with you.

If you went through all the previous steps correctly, then you gradually form the first stage of mastering intuitive nutrition. If characterized by despair, reduced self-esteem, and a feeling of inability to maintain another diet, go to the second stage of mindful eating - hyper consciousness at this stage, it is normal to pay increased attention to food and to be preoccupied with what, when, and how I eat, more than usual. You say - how is this different from dietary behavior? The fundamental difference is that dietary fixation on food consists of almost constant, anxiety, fears, and guilt. You are always afraid to break this or that rule, to eat the wrong thing, to make mistakes and be tormented, because you are surely mistaken, you are necessarily eating the wrong thing. You keep from doing anything all the time. In the second phase of intuitive nutrition, you do something completely different: constantly listen to yourself and ask questions: "Are you hungry? What do you want? This or that? Is it tasty to you? "And evaluate the level of your own satisfaction with this or that food. If this level is not high enough - this is not drama, not a disaster, not a violation of the rule. This is a training, valuable experience, and there is no personal guilt here - the food simply did not suit you. It happens.

At this stage, you begin to "reconcile with food," it ceases to be your constant enemy and rival. You do this by giving yourself permission to eat whatever you want. For many, this phase is experienced as frightening - a lot of people have never had such an experience in their life, so it is important to go through it at your own pace, comfortable for you, without haste.

At this stage, you will experiment a lot with food, trying it again, rediscovering the tastes forgotten due to many years of prohibitions. Paradoxically, it's a fact: allowing yourself to eat whatever you want, you may find that you don't like the products you dreamed of when they were banned. You may also find that it is difficult for you to stop when you are full, you continue to eat, having passed the saturation point. This is a normal process: restoration of contact with internal saturation signals follows after contact with hunger has been restored. It is important to follow this path step by step.

It is important to understand that hyper consciousness and the difficulties of managing eating behavior, even when you are already full, are not the final pattern that you seek to come to. This is a temporary stage in reconstructing your relationship with food as positive and free. Each of your food experiences ceases to be "right" or "wrong," each food becomes an instance in the collection of food experiences - not every instance of a true collector has the same value, which does not detract from the value of the collection as a whole.

This stage of mastering intuitive eating skills usually raises the most questions. Consider the most common of them.

Every Person Has "Priority Products"

This is the food that you choose most often in a situation where you need to have a bite, that food that is almost always "comfortable" for you (attention: this is about taste preferences, and not about the choice dictated by regular dietary considerations). Make a list of the food that you choose most often, and thoroughly stock up with the first five to six nominations in the list. Carry this food with you in a container for situations where hunger overtakes you on the road. This list is not permanent; it changes from time to time. The more accurately you listen to the signals of your own body, the more the list will change - you will proceed from the body's needs for certain substances without even realizing it.

"Hungry at the Wrong Time"

"I can't eat when I'm hungry, because I'm never hungry in the morning, later I run out to work. At work, I drink a couple of cups of coffee while I look through the accumulated mail, and so on until lunch. At lunch, I overeat, and until the evening, I remain with a feeling of heaviness from the stomach. "The task is to identify the moment when you are hungry accurately. If you don't feel like eating in the morning, hunger will catch you in 30 – 40 minutes. You will have to take food with you to be able to eat when you feel like it. Buy a large lunch box with compartments (even better for this purpose are boxes for sewing accessories, with many small compartments, each of which is closed with an individual lid). Put there what you like to eat in the morning - at least five different kinds of foods (yogurt, fruit, a little granola or cereal, small canapé sandwiches or cubes of cheese, ham, boiled chicken, small vegetables, nuts). It remains to get it at the moment when you are really hungry, and then I want to step back and talk about one strange cultural phenomenon that I have to observe while living at the junction of two different cultures.

The Dutch have the phenomenon of the "sacred sandwich" - whether it is a lecture at the university, an important high-level meeting, or a queue at the clinic - nothing will stop the Dutchman from getting a sandwich neatly packed in the morning and eating it decorously, without the slightest feeling of awkwardness. In the USA, according to my feelings, there is a rather powerful flow of awkwardness surrounding the "food taken from home." I can assume that this is somehow connected with the tradition of workers in factories and factories in the 1950s and later taking lunch with them. And no matter how skillful the wife is in cooking, no matter how delicious the home-made food, it is rare that any of the Western office workers will decide to "go with them" as opposed to a "business lunch" in a cafe so that there are no unnecessary associations. Parents in childhood also teach children about "eating indecently on the street." The maximum that children are allowed is ice cream.

The only recommendation I can give is to take responsibility for your food and your hunger. You have the inalienable right to eat if you are hungry. And if you are hungry on the way to work, then you have every right to satisfy this hunger. This is much more important than what others will think or say. Yes, I know that the road to work is not always very comfortable and conducive to food. But as soon as you say to yourself: "It's better to tolerate" - you take a step back, running again and again in the wheel of satisfying other people's needs at the expense of your own.

Shut down Negative Thoughts and Feel Right

I can't eat in public (in transport, on the go...).

Many compulsive eaters feel they have no right to eat, not only on the road but in any public place, except for a safe place at home. This is especially true for overweight people. How can they feel free to eat if they are already fat, ugly, and unattractive? This sensation has a direct connection with the global feeling "not entitled," characteristic of people with impaired eating behavior: not entitled to demand, ask, expect. Not entitled to say no.

There is no better way to start working with your satisfying the needs of others at the expense of your own than there is at a time when you have a need for it. Having won back from yourself and those around you, there is a right when and what you want, you can hope that the feeling that you are entitled will begin to spread to other areas of life. Usually, at first, this is manifested by flashes of sudden, unusual for your anger and irritation where previously you behaved modestly and unnoticed.

Do not be alarmed - this is how your autonomy is formed. The period of anger soon passes, giving way to the calm feeling "I have the right to do it," and this is a crucial stage not so much in the adjustment of nutrition as in the formation of a mature personality.

The theme of "give yourself the right" requires in-depth study, preferably in psychotherapy, if possible. You have no right to be hungry - what is it about in your personal past?

When working with these memories, with your resentment and anger, it is essential to continue to work with eating behavior, not to forget that these are two parallel, intensifying each other, processes. Being hungry, note that the fact that you are and going to eat doesn't affect at all and will not affect your relationship with other people. Perhaps this was in the past, but those times are past. Note also that it is unknown and entirely unimportant for other people whether you are eating now because you are hungry, or for other reasons. You deserve to notice your needs and meet them as they become available.

Fear of Hunger

G. Stein's book, The Confession of a Fat Psychiatrist, provides an instructive story. The author, the resident of the intensive care unit at a large American hospital, observes a patient who survived a plane crash. Being severely crippled, this person is in a particular device that evenly distributes pressure to all points of his body. This device slowly, delicately, but constantly changes the position of the human body relative to the earth, thus achieving the most uniform pressure distribution. Being under the influence of sedatives, most of the time, this patient calmly dozes off. Only once a day, when his body takes precisely the position in which it was at the time of the disaster, he wakes up and begins to scream heartbreakingly. Because the body remembers.

The body remembers other injuries inflicted on him. And strict diets are one of them. The experience of food restrictions leads to the fact that the feeling of hunger is associated with intense bodily discomfort, dizziness, and weakness, and a person who has such an experience naturally fears him. Fearing starvation, we start eating in advance to avoid it - and in the end, we eat more than necessary.

Tell yourself that you do not need to become so hungry. Develop for yourself a "mantra" that will help you cope with the attacks of this fear. It may be something simple, such as "I will eat as soon as I get hungry."

Feeling of Shame

"I can't eat in the presence of others" is a common problem. In this case, you have no difficulty in starting meals when you are hungry at home, but when you are at work, you are postponing and postponing a meal together with your colleagues. They saw your attempts to follow a particular diet, your overweight war, welcomed the victories, politely did not notice or let out sympathetic and sharp comments when the weight returned... You just can't eat in their presence anymore. Think about what exactly scares you in this. Speak privately with yourself in those fantasies in which your colleagues discuss behind your back your weight or the fact that you eat what you like. Now, remember that almost every person in the modern world experiences certain problems with food and body image, even thin people.

A sense of shame must necessarily be worked out in therapy, and preferably even in a group. In the meantime, you will do this work, consider the options - eat in your office, separately, or leave the place of work to eat.

I hear your grunts that you work where you have nowhere to go to eat. Sorry - this does not happen. At lunch, I often go to the park, a 5-minute drive from the clinic, where I sit on the grass and chew my salad, sandwich, or apple. Sometimes there is no time to go to the park - my colleagues and I set up a table and chairs right in the parking lot — not a park, but peace and quiet. Find a cozy place nearby - a clearing, a bench, and at least a curb with a view of something calm - greens, children playing on the playground, frolicking dogs, and go for a snack there.

Chapter 9: The Ninth Principle: Learn to Cope with Feeling Outside of Food

You have agreed to have dinner with a friend or girlfriend. You have a date or a family dinner. He still has two hours to go, but you want to eat now. Eating right now means not being able to enjoy your meal with friends or family. Do not eat - means to come to a meeting on legs bent from hunger and guaranteed to overeat. The essential thing in this and similar situations: you want to eat now, and not in two hours.

We return to the basics - there is, as soon as you feel hunger. That is - now. What is right now that will saturate you best, distracting from marvelous steaks in the restaurant where you go in two hours? Yeah, the remains of meat salad (yesterday's pasta, casseroles...) were nestled in the fridge. And exactly about them, you dreamed on the way from work? Excellent - get it. Just put yourself not your usual portion, but about a third or even a quarter. Eat until you just slightly satisfy your hunger, cut off the very top, so to speak. This is enough to live for two hours, and you will enter the restaurant hungry enough to eat what you want.

Find what most harmoniously suits your current needs, and eat just a little so that the hunger feeling is dulled, but preserved.

Do not "intercept" cookies, do not try to drown out the hunger for coffee - we often do this in order to pretend that we didn't eat anything at all - so we ran through the bridge, grabbed a maple leaf like the notorious goat from a fairy tale. If you allow yourself to stop and eat a little, but thoroughly and consciously, then you will not only put off your hunger - you will get the experience of respectful and careful handling of your own body and save yourself from the danger of moving to a restaurant.

This technique is called "hunger management" and can be used whenever you need it. In short - making a choice between the social situation and hunger right now, you make a decision. Or your hunger is strong enough to eat now, and then in a social situation, you will dispense with a cup of tea and small talk because you will not have time to get hungry. This choice is worth making if your hunger is really strong right now. Or you decide to dull the hunger a little with a small amount of food you desire. Then you will have the opportunity to enjoy food and chat at the same time. Your only task, making any choice, is to stop as soon as you are full at the main meal.

Another frequent complaint that I hear is that I get so involved in the work that I forget to eat, and when I come to, the feeling of hunger is so strong that I eat anything, overeat and suffer from pain in my stomach. This is especially affected by those who, it would seem, are in the most comfortable conditions for food - working at home. The solution, as usual, turns out to be very simple: be sure to cook yourself a meal early in the morning before you start. Put it in a container and put it on your desktop. No, do not take it to the kitchen because you will forget it there.

Lay on the table next to the computer. Then at the right moment, you can tell yourself - just a short pause, and I'll be back - and start eating right away. Write yourself a reminder on your phone, computer, and tablet that flashes every hour: "Hello! Are you hungry? How much? " Now, "It's time to eat!" But in the form of a question - you don't know when you are hungry. But now you can regularly check if you are hungry, and as soon as you feel hunger, you can satisfy it. And if, when you see a reminder, you will glance at the Hunger Scale and determine how hungry you are, then things will go faster.

"In Our Family, It Is Customary to Eat Everything Together"

What does this mean in practice? Different options are possible, for example: "Other family members express dissatisfaction if I eat separately," or "I'm anxious that if I postpone my meal until later, the children and husband will eat everything and I will remain hungry," or, perhaps, "It's hard for me to resist if everyone eats, but I don't."

Ask yourself why you are gathering together at the table every night, and why this is important to you. It is unlikely that you are united by food, communication - this is what is in the center. Nothing prevents you from enjoying communication with your family, even without a plate filled to the brim with food. You can eat earlier if you are hungry. You can put yourself a regular serving and set it aside for later if you are still not hungry. All this does not prevent you from sharing with your family a conversation about how the day went. If the family meal is very important for you, consider the following. Over time, as your experience as an intuitive eater increases, you can more accurately predict when you get hungry. In an hour or two, subtle bodily signals will tell you - you want to eat then. And if that doesn't match your life schedule, some fruit or a tiny sandwich will allow you too easily "put off your hunger." Give yourself time to ripen to this condition.

There is another nuance. The ability to eat separately from your family, "according to my desire," enhances the feeling of personal autonomy. And if in the relationship with husband/wife, parents, adult children, the topic of your autonomy is painful and unresolved (you are a "person without properties," without personal needs, you have no right to want), then your desire on when you need it will cause resistance on the other side. It is all the more important to defend this autonomy because insufficiently autonomous people are forced to seize their own negative emotions in order not to upset other people.

It is very important to understand that the more often and more accurately you respond to your body's call for food, the faster you develop the experience necessary to restore normal eating behavior.

Do not forget: eating for the wrong reasons will only give you the wrong results. As soon as one of the rules is violated, a feeling is formed that the entire system crashes, and overeating begins.

Chapter 10: The Tenth Principle: Give Yourself Grace, Practice Radical Self-Love

Exercise 1: "List of Priority Products"

Each of us has certain products that we tend to choose first when we are hungry. This list changes from month to month, from year to year, is replenished, or becomes shorter, but it always exists. Remember what food you are ready to eat always, everywhere, and it seems that you will never get tired of it? If you go to a restaurant with a buffet system, what exactly will you go with a plate in the first place - meat, cheese, desserts, and vegetables? If you are on a trip and live in a hotel where breakfast is offered to your room, what exactly do you miss most for breakfast - a glass of hot milk, your special flakes, cottage cheese? It's completely natural for the body to have priority products at every moment of time: it's not so much a matter of personal tastes,

Make a list of products that are your priority right now. Pay attention to the needs for yogurt of this particular producer, in the bread of this particular baking - these are not whims, this is really important.

For example:

1. Strawberry yogurt, "Chobani."

2. Roasted almonds.

3. Borodino bread.

Exercise 2: "Food with Me ... What Bothers Me?"

Imagine that tomorrow you need to take food with you for the whole day, so that the right foods are always at arm's length from you, at any time of the day.

What do you lack to do this? Need to buy the necessary products in the store? To cook something for the future? Buy a convenient container?

If you find that the obstacle is not a practical problem, but an emotional one - a feeling of shame and awkwardness that you have to eat in public or in a not very convenient place, imagine that tomorrow you will go to work, to school and to classes with children, in social institutions for business not alone - you will have a small child, no more than three years old, exactly like you in childhood. It is you who you will feed, and it is for him that you take food with you.

Exercise 3: Creating a Breeding Ground

Start creating at home, at work, in other places where you have to spend a lot of time, stocks of various food.

Free one shelf in a cupboard or refrigerator and warn family members or colleagues that your "special" products will lie on it. Glue a large, bright label on the shelf, such as Natasha's food, Dad's stocks. Arrange with your family that they can also create personal shelves for the products they need - this is a good reason to teach the whole family the basics of intuitive nutrition! First of all, stock up "priority" products from the list compiled during the previous exercise.

The Principle of Optimal Combination

Until now, all food has been divided for us according to the principles of "bad" (but contagion, desirable and tasty!) And "good" (but boring, tasteless and dull). To eat intuitively means to trust your body in that it is not disposed to harm yourself. Mother's milk always contains the ideal concentration of substances necessary for the baby - it is known that the milk of mothers of premature babies is more abundant in proteins, fats, and iron.

Studies confirm that if a person begins to consume vitamin C in amounts exceeding those necessary for the body, the body starts to actively remove excess vitamin C. With a lack of iron in food, the body absorbs more iron than usual. Thus, if you, at the time when you experienced real hunger, chose exactly the food that you wanted, this is the perfect combination.

The signs of the perfect combination are simple - this is exactly the food that you dreamed about, and by eating it, you feel physically good. If, after eating, you feel heaviness, bloating in your stomach, slight nausea, dissatisfaction, although you have eaten enough, there was a mistake, and the combination was not ideal.

For us, it's completely unimportant whether "good" is food or "bad." I know that this very moment often seems the most frightening, almost shocking: "If I am given free rein, I will eat some sweets!" In fact, as your natural and instinctive awareness of nutrition increases, you will intuitively refuse certain types of food, they will seem to you desperately tasteless - the body will protest against a bad attitude. Most often, the first on this list is, oddly enough, fast food.

Ask yourself: "If I had a magic wand that would give any food I wanted, what I would wish for?" The best combination is exactly the product or dish that you want to eat at the moment.

So far, you have regularly been practicing asking yourself the question, "Am I hungry now?" And "How hungry am I?" From now on, we will add to these questions one more, no less important: "What exactly do I want now?"

Eating exactly what you want at the moment means asking yourself before starting a meal, which meal will satisfy and saturate your body best? Much depends on what are the individual characteristics of your perception as a whole. Do you tend to think in pictures? The easiest way to try to imagine what the right dish looks like. If visual perception is not your strongest point, try to imagine the structure and taste that you now need.

So, crunchy or soft? Hot or cold? Salty or sweet? Spicy or fresh? The combination of these factors will lead you to the right dish. Cold, soft, sweet - yogurt, ice cream. Hot, soft, sweet - porridge. Elastic, spicy, hot - perhaps a steak or fried tofu? Allow yourself to play with different tastes, do not forget to realize what it is, what you are eating right now.

With the optimal combination found in your body, harmony comes from what you eat. You do not experience heaviness, heartburn, or other unpleasant sensations. This is a signal that the combination is found correctly. If the combination was wrong, do not despair, continue to analyze. It seemed like chicken, you chose fried chicken with potatoes, but did you feel the weight? Do you like chicken? Would it be the best combination of boiled chicken or Caesar salad?

If the best combination cannot be found - you want food that is objectively inaccessible, try to imagine the closest alternative - which could adequately replace the desired one? Often, when you start looking for an alternative, you find that you do not want to eat at all, and the desire for an unusual and inaccessible food was not a body signal, but an emotional experience.

When you master the skills described in this and the next chapters, at some point, you will find yourself in the Third stage of mastering intuitive nutrition - crystallization of the experience. At the crystallization stage, your intuitive eater, asleep before, begins to awaken. You got rid of dietary thinking, and you no longer need hyper consciousness in order to respond to your own hunger. You reconciled with the food, and it is no longer your enemy. For mastering the last skill, we will need materials from these following two chapters.

Chapter 11: The Eleventh Principle: Eat What Your Body Tells You To!

As a continuation of the tenth principle, we see that by agreeing to divide the food into "good" and "bad," we create a strange, distorted food industry with our own hands. In it, the concept of "tasty" - prepared from fresh and natural products, pleasing, delivering sensual pleasure - will change to the concept of "harmful" and "forbidden," so when they want to sell a product to us as "tasty," they'll necessarily add which, according to the manufacturer, symbolizes the temptation - chocolate, icing, and fat cream.

In fact, the food should be just delicious, pleasing, and nourishing. And "goodies" are not universal - what your body needs right now is tasty. If you want a marzipan cake, and you start spreading sugar-free jam on a dry cracker, you end up eating a packet of crackers and a jar of jam, overeat, you feel bad both physically and emotionally, but the "taste hunger" does not disappear - you need to want a marzipan cake still. And it will certainly "lie in wait" for you - visiting friends, at a birthday party, in a cafe, in a store at a discount at the checkout - and then you will not miss yours, and instead of one piece that you would eat then, it will be all yours - in vain, or something, you suffered and suffered. This does not say anything about your control - the strength of unmet need as a "salmon" makes you go upstream to spawn if you eat a marzipan cupcake at a time when you want it, voila! - The problem is resolved. The need is satisfied, it cozily and peacefully folds inside until the next time, and disaster does not happen.

Exercise: "How I Make Food Decisions"

1) Analyze and make a list of exactly how you make nutritional decisions - which primarily depends on what you will eat. For example:

a. Eat what is in the refrigerator;

B. Eat the rest from yesterday, or that threatens to deteriorate;

c. I buy in a cafe or make food in the dining room which is cheaper;

d. I watch what others eat and choose the same.

2) Remember the maximum possible number of situations and try to describe all the options. If you have a long experience in diets, then you have a lot of experience that you do not want. If you have food rules that force you to take food as carefully as possible to the detriment of your own body, you also have a lot of such experiences. This means that it may not be possible to understand what your body needs now immediately. It's okay - it's just a skill, and it can be developed.

Look at your list. Is there an item "Eat what I want at the moment"? No?

3) Then carefully cross out each of the items on your list and add this item: "I eat what I want at the moment." From now on, you will eat this and that only way.

The Search for Signals of Food Satisfaction

So far, we have practiced a key skill that is basic for the development of Intuitive Nutrition: the ability to start eating, feeling a certain, not very large, level of hunger. We also tried to evaluate the level of saturation that occurs as a result of food. Saturation is a physiological state, but the level of satisfaction from food is both physiological and psychological.

Remember what you ate recently. If you ate according to the principle of optimal combination, then you have a high level of satisfaction with food. This means that after eating, you are in a state of physiological comfort, and you feel how good your body is from what you eat. But not only. You are comfortable recalling the color, the smell of what you just ate, and you are pleased to recall the image of this dish, the circumstances of this meal.

It is difficult to achieve a high level of food satisfaction if you came home extremely hungry - your glass was almost empty - and hastily, unable to endure hunger anymore, ate right at the open door of the refrigerator, drowning in impatience. You can't achieve a high level of satisfaction with food even if you read, watched a movie, looked through email while eating. A high level of nutritional satisfaction requires not only the "right" food - the one you want right now but also a situation in which you can fully enjoy this food. Eating with a high level of nutritional satisfaction, you quickly notice how the amount of food needed for satiety is reduced.

Please note that levels of satiety and nutritional satisfaction may vary. In some cases, you can eat up to a high level of satiety - "full," the glass is almost full or completely full, but the level of food satisfaction – comfort and pleasure are low. This happens if you ate hastily, in uncomfortable circumstances, or not what you really wanted to eat. It may be the other way round: the saturation level is not very high, you ate a little, your glass remained half empty, but the satisfaction you eat is at its best.

Search for the Best Combination

How to determine what you want to eat right now? Try not to think in "terms of dishes," but in "terms of qualities" - hot, sweet, crumbly, buttery - perhaps buckwheat porridge with sugar and butter. Cool, sour, liquid - kefir or sour summer soup, or maybe iced tea with lemon?

Chapter 12: The Twelfth Principle: Making Peace with Your God-Given Shape

In modern culture, it is generally accepted that the body is not a harmonious, self-regulating system, but actually, an unbridled animal that must be kept in check and treated with all severity. Adding to this tyranny of unrealistic bodily perfection, are broadcast on the media.

The result of this is a hostile, negative attitude towards one's own body that can be "betrayed" at any time - not want to play sports or want forbidden food, and which, no matter how hard you try, does not meet the standards of glossy magazines.

The result is painful experiences of hatred of the body and bodily shame, which are often the cause of another attempt to go on a diet or go to the gym. Most of these attempts are doomed to failure, which causes even greater shame and even greater hatred. Therefore, the transition to an intuitive and informed diet is impossible without changing the attitude towards one's own body. The path to a harmonious life without diets and overload begins at the moment when you are able to accept your body now for what it is. Very often, the history of a negative attitude towards the body turns out to be so long that changes require effort and are not easy.

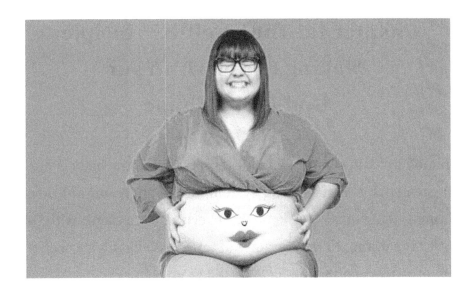

Where to start the path to positive self-acceptance? With three important things: cabinets, mirrors, and scales.

Cabinets

In the story that I will tell now, very many can recognize themselves. A young woman, completely falling under the description of the psychological profile of compulsive eaters, who is obese, loves shopping in addition to food. The girl has a great taste; she understands luxury brands, to a fault. On one of the trips to the same places, the girl discovers the Dream Dress. The dress was made by the Fashion Designer, and it costs, with all the discounts and sales of the rest of the collection, 500 dollars. A rather big sum for a girl, but she wants to love herself and not something there? And can you afford it? Dress bought!

Of course, it is 2 sizes smaller than necessary and does not converge on the chest and abdomen. "After all, I will ever lose weight!" So from the subject of pampering myself, my beloved, the dress becomes a punishment, a sword of Damocles hanging over our heroine, whom she meets every time, opening the closet. "You are my disappointment," says Dress. "You still haven't lost weight and can't put me on to a party ... In all likelihood, you can never put me on." Because I must be earned."

The girl did not need to be beautiful; she needed a distant, beautiful goal, which this Dress remarkably symbolized. In the process of psychotherapeutic work, she began to sell branded things of an unrealistic size for herself at an online flea market. Most of all, she was struck by the fact that the income from these sales amounted to little monies. Although she sold things very cheaply, she was hoping to get rid of them as quickly as possible. "Why did I torment myself so?" She asked herself thoughtfully, talking about it.

How many clothes are hanging in your closet? If you have a long experience of fighting with your own body, then the typical answer is at least three. One is the size that you are wearing now. The second is clothing in case you get better. The third is clothing in case you lose weight, which you cannot wear right now, but hope to start wearing in the very near future. Many weight loss programs encourage customers to keep their "slim" clothes - it is believed that this motivates the program participant to adhere to a nutrition plan and training. Ask yourself how you feel when looking inside such a cabinet. The answer will be sadness, dissatisfaction, despair. The presence of clothes in a closet that you cannot fit in that size will cause an alarm that often leads to the result of overeating.

Imagine opening your closet in which your clothes hang every day. There are a lot of clothes hanging in which you cannot fit in, since they are too small for you. There are clothes that fit your size, but you don't like it very much - you're tired a lot, there are a lot of black clothes or clothes in dark colors. Many things do not fit together - because you don't make wardrobe choices, buying random things while waiting for you to lose weight and buy the clothes that you really like.

Now imagine that you open a closet with clothes that fit your size. You can put on each of the things there. Colors and styles reflect your condition, mood. How do you feel looking in this closet? How do these feelings affect your condition throughout the day?

Inventory Task

Go through the closet in which your clothes are hanging, and get rid of all the ones that do not fit you in size. Make a list of what's left. Plan what you are missing for the wardrobe to be full, and replenish it with clothes of your current size. The most frequent reactions to this task are complaints about the lack of money for purchases and the lack of clothing stores for large people. Both that and another is a form of resistance - large clothing also exists.

Scales

Scales are medical devices invented to measure a person's weight. In modern culture, scales have become an instrument that supports and enhances bodily dissatisfaction. People, preoccupied with their weight, attribute to the scales incredible power to determine whether they will have a "good" today or a "bad" today. Many people often weigh themselves several times during the day, hoping to see a decrease in numbers, go to the toilet specially or remove jewelry before standing on the scales.

Using the scale as a tool to control nutrition is doomed to failure. Most people, noticing weight gain, exhibit some signs of distress: increased anxiety, panic attacks, decreased mood, and this significantly increases the risk of overeating. It would seem that if the scales show a decrease in weight, this should improve the condition and provide support. However, many people say that when the scales show the desired numbers, the alarm only increases: it's scary not to keep what you've achieved, I want to reward myself for finally getting the desired result, I get the feeling that "you can eat safely today, since everything is fine with weight "- and this launches new cycles of diet and overeating.

In addition, it should be remembered that scales are an extremely inaccurate tool for determining body size. Muscles are heavier than fat. Those who begin to regularly move actively notice weight gain by numbers on the scales, while endurance and well-being improve. A woman's weight varies depending on the phase of the menstrual cycle, depending on the level of hormones.

If your goal is a harmonious relationship with your own body, then the best way out is to completely get rid of the scales in the house and stop weighing.

At the same time, you will maintain an understanding of whether you are gaining weight or losing weight - from the feeling of how the clothes are sitting on you.

The decision to get rid of weights is an important step towards self-acceptance. This is a recognition that the numbers on the scales cannot serve as a regulator of the level of your self-esteem. Much more important is how you feel about work, close relationships, about your hobbies, and interests.

Mirrors

Another important step in the process of self-acceptance involves working with mirrors. Many people with bodily shame completely avoid mirrors both at home and elsewhere. Others use the mirror to criticize themselves ruthlessly. The purpose of working with a mirror is to learn to look at yourself with a calm and accepting look, rather than criticizing and hating. The path to a positive body image lies through the transshipment point of a neutral, non-judgmental attitude. Do not try to change annihilating comments to approving ones immediately - it just won't work.

At this stage, it is important to use every opportunity to look at yourself in the mirror. Looking in the mirror, try to simply describe what you see, avoiding any ratings - both negative and positive. "The belly is round, protruding, muscular calves and rounded hips" - imagine that you are describing your body to a scientist studying the structural features of a white (or black, or brown) race person. Explore the body, get acquainted with it - this is the basis for the subsequent good relationship.

Do not forget that the interpretation of the complete figure as ugly is absent in many cultures and societies. I recall in this connection to another story.

A young Dutchman with morbid obesity and a very difficult childhood experience, in which he learned all the lessons correctly and developed exactly the traits that are necessary to compensate for the traumatic situation in the family, turned out a very respectable, modest, extremely persistent intellectual achievement perfectionist who knows how to dissociate in relationships and not achieve intimacy effectively. Suffering significant excess weight already in his teens and having received from classmates everything that full teens receive in the framework of our culture, he forever realized for himself that "but he is smart." He received an excellent education and became a rather successful lawyer - panic attacks prevented a shining speech in court, but outside the walls of the courtroom, the young man achieved excellent results in the conduct of business. He considers himself ugly and categorically unattractive. Two attempts to build relationships with girls end in failure - he is too distant, unable to open up, unable to trust and believe that he is loved. Relations are broken.

Finally, in search of a relationship for which his detachment is not a hindrance, he chooses a girl from Thailand who practically does not speak Dutch. Communication in a language that is not native to both, English, provided a sufficient sense of security, and the young man does not run away from relationships in the first three months. And then he discovers that his girlfriend finds him sexually and physically attractive. For him, this is an alien mail message; he cannot immediately destroy the negative opinions about his own unattractiveness, but he cannot but believe her. And then the young man experiences a deep cultural shock - when the girl answers the question of what exactly seems physically attractive to him in him - your fullness. In Thailand, she says, a complete (fat) person is considered beautiful, handsome, and worthy of respect.

In this story, the young lawyer's belief in his ability to be not only smart but also attractive, developed very slowly and gradually. It doesn't happen in another way. In the process of doing this work, you will, again and again, break into criticism of the body. Once this happens, stop the mirror exercise, even if you have just started it.

As your experience with the mirror builds up, your quality of life will improve. You will no longer be shocked by the way you look in photographs or video shooting - a good acquaintance with your own body will help. Gradually, a neutral and calm attitude towards how you look will replace criticism and hatred. This will lead to an increase in confidence and self-esteem.

Many at this stage note that despite the fact that a neutral or positive image of the body can be easily kept at home, going beyond it still brings great stress, especially if the weight is objectively large. The views and comments of other people will attack you if, from the point of view of the generally accepted culture of thinness, you look like a big man. Do not forget that this is a manifestation of the hatred that such people have for their own bodies. Your increased self-esteem hurts them, pointing to your body and the acute experience of their imperfection.

Nevertheless, you will probably notice that negative thoughts about the body revolve in your head over and over again and that you need to work more actively with them to change relationships with the body. Negative thoughts about the body are often learned in early childhood or adolescence. The randomly dropped comments of parents and relatives, comparisons with other, slimmer or more attractive children, competition between children in the family and competition between classmates for the title of the most attractive, as well as acquaintance with the world of glossy magazines - all this creates the basis for the formation of a constant stream of negative thoughts about the body.

These thoughts are psychologically "toxic" and are responsible for the constantly high background of anxiety, decreased mood, eating "breakdowns," and are involved in the development of severe eating disorders such as bulimia, anorexia, and compulsive overeating.

The problem of dissatisfaction with one's body has become so widespread and relevant among young people aged 16–25 that in the USA, a special Body Education Program was developed for college and university students. One of the interventions undertaken in this program was the introduction of Fat Talk Free Weeks, a period free from "bold conversations." Launched in 2008, this five-day awareness-raising and positive body attitude programs are now held annually internationally. Within 5 days of the week, any phrases like "I'm so fat!" "Oh, you look cool! Lost weight?" "I need to go on a diet," "With that weight, you shouldn't put it on," "Does my ass look fat?"- It's simply forbidden. At the same time, seminars and lectures on the destructive influence of the "ideal of thinness" are held.

The result of this program after 8 months was that 53% of the women who participated in it no longer felt the overwhelming and fundamental effect of weight on their own lives. 48% of women who had previously felt "fat" almost daily, either completely ceased to feel that way, or the periods of such experiences were significantly reduced. More than half of the program participants who reported that thoughts and feelings about weight and appearance prevent them from focusing on their studies reported a significant improvement at the end of the program.

What does this mean? Words have a much greater effect on us than we are used to thinking. And when you, even flirting a little and hoping to get a rebuttal, ask your girlfriend or partner: "Am I not fat in this dress?" - You are hurting yourself.

In the presence of signs of disturbed eating behavior, getting rid of negative thoughts about the body is a mandatory step, without which the sustainable establishment of a positive and harmonious attitude to food is doomed to failure.

The 4-Step Transformation Assignment

Write down a few negative thoughts about the body that visit you most and annoy you the most. This can be an experience concerning a separate part of the body ("I hate my fat thighs") or the whole appearance in general ("I look like a disgusting cow"). Choose one of them to transform.

You can carry out the transformation yourself, but working in a group or in a pair is ideal for this. If, while reading this manual, it occurred to you that you want to recommend it to someone from friends, acquaintances, or colleagues, this person will be a good candidate for such a job.

Stage 1 – Apology

Say aloud your negative thought about the body: in the mirror to yourself, to another member of your couple or group (there can be as many people as you like in the group) as if you were speaking to him and not talking about yourself. For example, "I hate your fat thighs," "I feel sick of your blurry figure."

Then, after a pause, also out loud, apologize for what you said. Choose the words that you find suitable in order to ask for forgiveness in such a situation.

If you performed this part of the exercise alone, note your own feelings when performing the first and second parts. If you worked in a couple or group, ask the partner in this work to tell you how he felt when you voiced your thoughts and when you apologized, and then share your feelings.

Stage 2 – Confrontation

Ask yourself: why do you think thin hips are better than full hips? Where did this idea come to you from when it first appeared in your head? Who told you that this is so, and not otherwise? Ask yourself this question every time it comes to your mind.

Changing internal beliefs does not happen on the same day, but regular questions to yourself on this topic successfully "undermine their credibility."

Stage 3 – Stop

To have or not have negative thoughts about the body in your own head is a matter of personal choice. If you have them, then you allow them to appear. The flow of negative thoughts about the body can be stopped; the negative image of the body can be changed for the better. Despite the fact that this is not easy for anyone, the result is worth the effort.

Visualization Exercise

Sit or lie down, find a comfortable position for the body. Close your eyes, and remember the most recent negative thought about the body that visited you. Now imagine how this statement appears on the computer screen - as if it were being printed. Press the delete button! We print a more positive (or neutral) statement that does not hurt or devalue you, for example: "I am saddened by the way my hips look now, but we are working on it." While finding a positive or neutral statement can be a daunting task, continue to formulate options until the one you find suits you completely.

Stage 4 – Decoding

The last stage of working with negative thoughts about the body is based on the idea already expressed earlier that worries about an insufficiently perfect body or "wrong" weight always conceal other, deeper problems of relationships with the world. Try to decipher what is hidden behind experiences like "I have a terrible, ugly saggy stomach" or "I'm so loose and fat." What does it mean for you that other people will see or consider you "fat," "a man with a fat belly," "wide-hipped"?

Does this mean that you are scared of the idea of attracting attention to yourself, and therefore you hesitate to wear bright clothes or take pictures? Or are you afraid of being rejected and, therefore, avoiding intimacy, and being overweight is a good excuse not to go on dates? You may be avoiding graduate meetings, explaining this as "loss of form," but in fact you're scared that everyone will see how the former excellence student and medalist did not become anyone other than the wife and mother of three children, instead of making a bright and an enviable career? Start spinning this mental spiral back (you can do it in writing).

What is the most typical negative thought about the body that comes to your mind when you look in the mirror, go to a party, interview for a new job?

1. I am too fat; I look disgusting.

What does it mean to look disgusting, what consequences will it lead to if you still decide to leave the house?

2. I have no right to dress beautifully. I cannot wear a red dress.

What happens if you still wear a red dress and leave the house?

3. Everyone will look at me, pay attention.

And what will it do to you?

4. It is unbearable.

So, the idea that "I am too fat" hides the idea that attracting the attention of other people is unbearable and causes a feeling of great anxiety. Will this sensation disappear if you lose weight? No, it will stay with you because it is not related to weight. Weight is just a cover.

Your negative thoughts about the body - never just about the body - they carry an important encrypted message about those problems that really concern you and largely determine your lifestyle and behavior. To face these problems is always unpleasant, but, ultimately, necessary to improve the quality of life.

Conclusion

Problems with eating behavior are always a "signboard" behind which deeper life problems are hidden. To identify and work out the internal conflicts that have been "stored" in us from early childhood is a large-scale and difficult task that can be solved when you have the resources to do this: strength, time, and motivation. And they appear when you stop endlessly worrying about whether you can eat this cake and what number the scales will show today, be afraid to go to the party, because there will be a lot of delicious food and you will lose your diet, or because you are not enough to look good in this outfit, once again with annoyance and longing there is a tasteless, but healthy food, dreaming of completely different dishes and angry all over the world that you are so unhappy - even the simple right to eat what you want is deprived!

In fact - you can eat everything, you can always, and you can eat everywhere. After all, food is only one of the many pleasures in the world. Remember that your body is an amazing gift, an obedient and faithful servant, the most reliable partner in all your endeavors.

The body does not refuse and continues to serve you, no matter what. Show mercy to it. Give thanks to it. The feeling of having a full life found in response to what they have is what makes a person happy. And you deserve happiness - I know that for sure. And I thank you in advance on behalf of your body and my own.

Sincerely yours,

Ashley Brain.

Made in the USA
Middletown, DE
14 June 2022